LIMITS

THE KEYSTONE OF EMOTIONAL GROWTH

John E. Poarch, M.D., F.A.P.A.

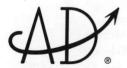

Accelerated Development Inc.
Publishers
3400 Kilgore Avenue
Muncie, IN 47304-4896

LIMITS: The Keystone of Emotional Growth

Technical Development: Tanya Dalton
                          Marguerite Mader
                          Sheila Sheward

Library of Congress Cataloging-in-Publication Data

Poarch, John E., 1935-
    Limits : the keystone of emotional growth / John E. Poarch
        p.   cm.
    Includes bibliographical references and index.
    ISBN 1-55959-020-3
    1. Self-actualization (Psychology)   2. Self-control.   I. Title
    BF637.S4P62   1990   90-82966
    155.2--dc20

LCN: 90-82966

Accelerated Development Inc.
Publishers
3400 Kilgore Avenue
Muncie, IN 47304-4896
Toll Free Order Number 1-800-222-1166

TO ALL PEOPLE WHO RISK HONESTY
IN SPITE OF DOUBT AND INSECURITY,
AND TO THE FUTURE, OUR CHILDREN.

ACKNOWLEDGEMENTS

As a child I knew that my mother's dream was for me to become a minister. I preached impassioned hell and damnation sermons to the bedroom mirror or to the chickens, but in a flash the evangelist could convert himself to Captain Marvel, Superman; or I might suddenly decide to play at being a grand farmer with match box barns and huge fields, surrounded by string and twig fences. As a psychiatrist I have treated more than a few ministers. If it counts to minister to ministers, perhaps my mother's dream did indeed come true.

My father was too busy worrying about feeding and clothing his family to be very concerned with what I might become. He was poor, as money measures a person, but he was among the wealthiest of men, in terms of honesty and integrity. Although he influenced my life directly for less than sixteen years, because of his death from a coronary when I was a teenager, his example has shaped me more than that of any man. He taught me that if you are not honest, whatever else you achieve is of reduced value, or has little genuine meaning. I believe it is impossible to be absolutely honest with ourselves and the world at all times, but the critical difference lies in how hard we try to live by that ethical standard. My dad tried hard.

In time I decided that the solution for all of the problems of mankind was education. I determined to attain as much as I possibly could. In the twenty four years of formal education required to become a psychiatrist, I grew keenly aware and extremely appreciative of excellence in teaching. Some teachers, like Socrates and Plato, continue to teach infinite generations by means of their writings. Such contemporaries as Carl Sagan and Stephen Hawking are so impressive that I predict they also will continue teaching many generations. A feeling of reverence accompanies my reading the works of certain teachers who have educated me through their writings. Among those on my personal Honor Roll are the following:

Sigmund Freud—For the basic framework upon which has been built the psychiatry of today.

Eugen Bleuler—For his elaborate description of the four "A's": ambivalence, autistic thinking, looseness of association, and inappropriate affect.

Anna Freud—For her teachings about therapy of children and human defenses.

Freida Fromm-Reichmann—For her teachings about therapy of severely regressed patients.

Margaret Mahler—For her teachings about separation-individuation.

The latter three members of the roll would make more than adequate transference mothers for all involved in the mental health professions. By means of transference, we transfer feelings originally focused toward our mother onto other people including teachers.

Rene Spitz—For his wonderful teachings about early infancy.

Harry Stack Sullivan— For his teachings about the process of human interaction.

John Bowlby— For his teachings about the pain of separation.

Erik Erikson— For his teachings about phases of emotional development.

My Honor Roll among those who taught me in person includes:

Eugene Pumpian-Mindlin, M.D.—Who was a mentor for most residents who trained under him.

C. V. Ramana,—Who taught me not to settle for blaming as a substitute for phenomenological understanding.

Gordon Deckert, M.D.—In my third year of medical school while taking an elective to learn hypnosis under his tutelage, I complained to him of the boring, poorly organized course in psychiatry. Imagine my amazement when in my fourth year, Dr. Deckert volunteered to teach our course. It was extraordinarily organized, entertaining, and so informative that my class achieved higher average scores in psychiatry than any other subject. He was soon to become departmental chairman and is a pioneer in making the teaching of psychiatry to medical students a primary task of senior faculty rather than a minor chore assigned to the most junior faculty. Medical students at the University of Oklahoma have performed far above the national average on examinations in psychiatry for many years.

Povl Toussieng, M.D.,—For teaching me the critical difference between experiencing a hopeless feeling as an empathic communication from the patient rather than a diagnostic judgement.

My teachers who took the risk of being harmed in the hope of being helped were my patients. This book is evidence that their teachings were enormously significant to me. The privilege to treat people through psychotherapy provides the unique gratification of participation in growth rather than just observing it. I often say, "It is like getting to be a part of the flowers blooming rather than just observing." I am very grateful.

My family was at greatest risk, at least until the children were out of the home. They were and are among my best teachers; my wife, Anita, my sons, David and John, and my daughter, Maria. They would unanimously attest that I am a demanding and difficult student.

The psychiatric residents whom I have taught, and now teach, have taught me much in turn. Beyond this they continue to inspire, stimulate, and challenge me. It is also ever rejuvenating. Just as it is with my children, sheer delight is when they point out something I have missed or do not know. Progress depends on those students who eventually out-do their teachers.

I also appreciate my enduring and supportive secretary, Donna Rutherford, in spite of her promise to terminate her employment should I write another book before adjusting to an office word processor. Gladys Lewis gets credit for red marking the manuscript again and again, in spite of my wailing. It finally became a presentable semblance of English clarity and usage because of her able editorial assistance.

June , 1990   John E. Poarch

TABLE OF CONTENTS

DEDICATION .... **iii**

ACKNOWLEDGEMENTS .... **v**

INTRODUCTION **1**

SECTION I   ESSENTIAL CONCEPTS **5**

1. PLEASURE/PAIN PRINCIPLE **7**

2. MATURATION **11**
Blame 12
Overprotectiveness 13
No 15
Goodbye 16
Ambiguity 17

3. THE DYNAMIC STRUGGLE **19**

4. STRESS **23**

SECTION II: TRADITIONAL CLASSICS **27**

5. DEPENDENCY **29**
Emotional Dependency 30

6. AGGRESSION **33**

7. SEX AND INTIMACY **41**
Women Without Desire 44
We Relate the Same Sexually as Socially 45

SECTION III: SETTING LIMITS **49**

8. TIME **51**
Behavioral Communication 52

9. LIMITS **55**

10. RULES **59**
Allowances and Money 63
Telephone 64

11. OVERSTIMULATION **67**
Bribes 70
Danger 71
Overstimulation in the Pain Center 74

12. CONSEQUENCES **77**
School Discipline 83
Crime 84

13. ABOUT DATING, DRINKING, CARS, AND COLLEGE **85**
Drinking 87
Cars 88
College 89

SECTION IV: CLOSURE: ULTIMATE LIMITS **91**

14. LETTING GO **93**

15. SEPARATION **97**
Loss 98

REFERENCES **110**

INDEX **113**

ABOUT THE AUTHOR **117**

INTRODUCTION

When in his early teens my younger son, now a chemical engineer, remarked with profound sincerity, "Ya know, you should write a book. It ought to be called *Limits*."

"Well John, this is it!"

After reading one of my articles about marriage, my daughter, who was sixteen at the time, exclaimed, "No fluff. All meat, no salad. Needs more salad!" This statement perhaps best describes my style. In well over fifty thousand sessions of treating patients by use of medical psychotherapy, my repeated statements have become quite brief and without "fluff," my own limits and resulting discipline. A reliable structure for setting limits and administering consequences is essential to healthy emotional growth as well as for clear communication. This book will provide a framework for setting limits which is based on sound theory. Understanding ourselves and others requires such a structure so that we can have some idea of whether we are progressing, standing still, or going backwards regarding emotional growth and development.

My involvement with this book began at the emotional level of a participant in the process of family interaction. Intense stress was related to the required adjustment to the unusual socioeconomic success relative to my beginnings. Working through the resulting problems has contributed immensely to the ideas contained in these pages. I am a sharecropper's last child, and had seven older brothers and one sister; four are now deceased. My mother was nearly forty-four and my father was forty-nine when I was born. I have also shared in rearing three children quite successfully. The intense desire to please them and the painful doubt I experienced when a firm "No" was required was a major motivating factor toward my work on the issue of *Limits*. Fortunately, I was developing and testing the framework contained herein as they were growing-up. As adults, they all continue to delight and amaze me. All performed extremely well in their studies and in extracurricular activities, including sports. All proceeded to college with academic scholarships. My two sons have now graduated and have excellent employment with promising futures. My daughter is now in college.

But I also approach this book with the feelings of a professional practitioner of psychotherapy who helps people set limits in order that emotional growth can occur. *LIMITS* is a product of twenty years of psychotherapy practice: a career of observation and study with regard to this issue as it relates to the growth and development of individuals, groups, and nations.

Since emotional growth may continue until death, the book is global in usefulness. The book will be especially helpful to parents, teachers, teens, and those involved in mental health fields. It also has ramifications for the legal and educational systems. Those involved in setting limits and administering consequences for society, such as policemen, attorneys, judges, and legislators, can better understand the phenomena that result in criminality. *LIMITS* can promote understanding of repeating acts of crime immediately upon release from prison or just after termination of parole. The book can help educators understand why parents come forth quickly threatening a lawsuit when the school makes an attempt to deal with a serious behavior problem in a youngster. I wish I could have known what I am conveying here when I was a teen, a young parent, and in my early professional life.

For the most part, this book is made up of statements made to patients as the topics arise during the course of psychotherapy. At times it may sound as if I am speaking to a teenager, or an adult of any identity; more commonly, I am addressing the patient as parent or using examples of parent-child interaction to promote understanding.

The "Essential Concepts" of Section I includes the core hypothesis upon which my theory of limits is based. This is contained in Chapter 1 and explains how we must increase our tolerance for stimulation in the pain center of the brain in order to be able to tolerate more stimulation in the pleasure center which correlates with emotional growth. Chapter 2 will convey ways by which we can tell which direction our personal energies are leading us in the maturity/immaturity continuum. In Chapter 3 I will show how it is necessary to always struggle against tendencies toward overprotectiveness in order to increase our tolerance for emotional discomfort and thus develop. In Chapter 4 we learn that by increasing our tolerance for stimulation we can automatically increase our tolerance for stress and thereby reduce tendencies toward severe mental disturbance.

"Traditional Classics" of Section II are those areas of psychological development commonly delineated by mental health care professionals. These must be dealt with time and again throughout our lives. Contrary to popular belief, emotional maturity is achieved through overcoming our fear of our own dependency, aggression, and sexuality, not by increasing or decreasing our amounts. The more that we increase our tolerance for stimulation the less we fear our feelings and our impulses in all three areas.

When reading the chapter on *"Limits,"* in Section III, my wife enthusiastically remarked, "Now we are getting to the g-o-o-d part." Anyone who has trouble setting limits will find this section helpful. Although each chapter will stand alone, one needs to read the chapters in sequence in order to maximally understand the practical application of the basic theory. My intention is to show how setting limits and administering consequences can increase tolerance for all stimuli in both parent and child. The parent-child paradigm will apply equally well to any authority-subordinate relationship. *Limits* and consequences are essential for emotional growth to occur.

Section IV is about letting go, good-bye, and the ultimate goodbye which is death. Ideally, emotional growth results in our being able to let go, face goodbyes appropriately, and accept the fact that aging and death are inevitable.

As families, or as a nation, if we cheat on our taxes, throw trash out car windows, refuse to live within our means, or control what we put in our mouths, we cannot expect to be very useful in helping our children when they need assistance with their controls. In our society a glut of overstimulation and infantalization is due to overprotection. The United States has been a culture of intense competition and achievement. We have had such rapid success in our short history that we now see the evidence of overstimulation. In our child rearing practices, our legal system, and our government, overprotectiveness is producing stagnation and often regression. If we do not turn the system toward the direction of more clear limits and consequences, the natural course of events will lead increasingly to more destructive behavior which will force us to change or perish. The choice is ours.

I do not know of previous unified theory of limits. By unified, I mean one that is consistent with anatomy, neurochemistry, and current concepts of psychological growth and development. Students and practitioners in my profession search for a practical theory. Patients long for such a guide and individuals test limits for relief from overstimulation. I know the theory works. I developed, practiced, and tested the theory in this book in my private practice. It is also quite teachable, being applicable for private psychotherapists and psychiatric residents whom I supervise. Behavioral scientists must strive to achieve a theory of limits that is as reliable as the laws of physics, whether it be this theory, extensions of it, or a new one. Such an achievement is not out of the realm of possibility and it might save mankind from self destruction through misuse of knowledge. Limits and resulting discipline could have prevented Three Mile Island and Chernobyl. The more power man develops, the greater the need for *LIMITS*.

SECTION I

ESSENTIAL
CONCEPTS

CHAPTER 1

PLEASURE/PAIN PRINCIPLE

According to Freud's (1924) pleasure principle we seek pleasure and avoid pain. This hypothesis does not account for growth through conscious choice. We cannot grow by indulging ourselves. Growth could only occur by coincidence when events in our lives, such as loss, cause unavoidable emotional discomfort. This chapter sets forth an alternative theory which allows for growth by choice.

In my view, a very dramatic and important distinction exists between physical pleasure and pain versus emotional pleasure and pain. In the excellent book, *Molecules of the Mind*, (1987) Jon Franklin referred to the human brain being wrapped around the mammalian brain which is wrapped around a reptilian brain, and shows that each brain is a slave to the previous one. Only the human can grow emotionally to the extent that what we feel doesn't determine how we act. The most common example I can think of is getting out of bed in the morning when it is certainly not what we feel like doing. This chapter will discuss how we can promote actions independent of those which we feel like doing. In the rest of the book, I will be referring only to emotional pleasure/pain. I think of us humans as having a pleasure center and a pain center in our brain, much like in lower animals. Since the early research of Heath et al. (1954) and Olds(1956) much has been accomplished but our understanding in man remains incomplete (Wise & Rompre, 1989). For theoretical purposes we may consider that all pleasureful feelings stimulate the pleasure center, so whether we are referring to success, achievement, intimacy (including sexual excitement), freedom, or childlike anticipation, all of these stimulate the same focus in the brain. A confirming example might be a student making an "A" on an important examination resulting in a sexual dream the night after the results are obtained. Similarly, all negative or distressing feelings are a result of stimulation of the pain center. Whether we are referring to sadness, confusion, insecurity, doubt, fear, or any one of the dysphoric array of feelings, they all push the same button.

Emotional growth concerns increasing our tolerance for stimulation in these centers. By this I mean progressively resetting the alarms, as we would thermostats, so that we can tolerate higher highs and lower lows without losing control of our behavior. We cannot stand a greater intensity of stimuli in one center than the other. Expressed in a numerical analogy, if one could only tolerate a negative five then the tolerance in the pleasure center would be a positive five. I certainly do not mean to imply that there is a payback system, but only that the person who cannot stand much discomfort also cannot stand much real pleasure. Certain chemicals such as drugs and alcohol can turn off the alarms and this may help one understand habituation and addiction (Kornetsky, 1988; Izenwasser & Kornetsky, 1989).

The original alarm settings are determined by the people with whom we live when we are small children; that is, the signals are a matter of conditioning. A set of parents will have relatively the same settings, otherwise one partner would make the other too anxious and the relationship would be terminated long before any prospect of marriage arose. The parents whose settings are very low will condition their children's settings to be also very low. An obvious example might be the difference between a mother who responds to some mud on her child as though it is a matter of life and death, as opposed to the one who responds with little or no dismay.

I believe that humans have the potential for natural, unimpeded growth, just as flowers and trees respond to nature's force. But fear gets in the way and frustrates our natural tendencies. Through our behavior, we consciously seek comfort or sameness, but unconsciously seek risk, that which will foster growth. This may not be reflected at all in our thoughts and feelings. The criminal is afraid but unconsciously desires to be stopped. The person behaving in any immature manner wishes the behavior not to be accommodated. If I do not insist that the patient with intense feelings of inadequacy keep his/her bill current, I am behaving as though that person is in fact inadequate and thus I cannot help him/her. Regardless of what words or feelings occur in our sessions, my behavior is telling him/her that indeed he/she does not measure up and is not expected to pay on time as everyone else does.

I do not believe that we can force ourselves to tolerate more pleasure. We will "blow it" every time. We may act in such a way as to provoke a friend or mate if the closeness becomes threatening. We may arrive late, lock our keys in the car, have an accident, or get a speeding ticket. If we delude ourselves with drugs or alcohol, substances which turn off the alarm in the pleasure center, we will eventually lose control of their use.

I do believe that we can force ourselves to tolerate more pain. To do so requires that we do what we intellectually know to do no matter how we feel. It does not mean that we turn off or deny our feelings. It does mean letting the baby cry when that is the last thing on earth we want to do. It means being honest in spite of the fact that someone's feelings are going to be hurt, but not in order to hurt. It means administering consequences to my child for breaking rules, even when the child is responding as though she or he will never love me again. It means not lending money to a relative who is always in a desperate predicament. It means being straight with myself and my mate even though I feel certain it will result in divorce.

Only if I take the ultimate risk will I discover that the result is the opposite of what I fear. By taking increasing risk which leads progressively toward the ultimate risk, I can and will reset the alarm in my pain center. I believe this is consistent with biology, anatomy, and physiology. This will eventually lead me to be able to tolerate more and more of life's losses, which Judith Viorst (1986) called necessary, and our own aging and mortality. This will free us to be more and more real. We can then enjoy all of life's fruits to the maximum. We will, by this means, no longer be complete slaves to our more primitive brains. The increased tolerance also will be passed directly to our progeny since their conditioning will be different to this same degree.

I shall refer to this concept again and again when I discuss the subject of limits. This theoretical construct is the core of the growth and development model and all the ideas in all the chapters are consistent with it.

In summary the Pleasure/Pain principle asserts that emotional growth is achieved through gradually increasing our tolerance for stimulation in the pain center of the brain. Through enduring those discomforts which come our way and by forcing ourselves to tolerate more discomfort by such means as being honest or saying "No" when that is absolutely the last thing we wish to do, we can increase our tolerance for pain. Observations show that this will automatically increase the tolerance in the pleasure center by a corresponding degree.

CHAPTER 2

MATURATION

Maturity and immaturity exist on the same continuum. The more mature people are the less is their tendency to blame, be overprotective, or avoid arguments. The less difficulty they have saying or accepting "No," corresponds with less difficulty in saying goodbye. The more able they are at facing anything related to injury or death, the better they tolerate being frustrated, and the more their tolerance for ambiguity, doubt, and uncertainty. Note that all of these factors are related to emotional discomfort. The ability to tolerate positive feelings such as intimacy, freedom, excitement, and success correlates directly with our tolerance for emotional discomfort. The mature person reacts to fear with sublimation, as exemplified by the physician who confronts the fear of his/her own injury and death, the policeman or the minister who faces the fear of losing control of impulses, and even the psychiatrist who deals with his/her own fear of craziness.

The opposite then follows: the more immature people are, the more they lean toward the above tendencies. Of course, people can learn to cover-up these traits in order to hide or defend against their lack of maturity. For example, they say, "By Golly! If other people can do it, so can I," while turning off feelings in order to take the risk. Imagine a person on a roller coaster with eyes tightly closed and the individual's entire body tensed with a death grip on the safety bar.

To give you a practical example of mature versus immature, look at the reaction of a relatively mature person to injury. He or she will not be terribly outraged or vindictive, nor become a very demanding, hostile, whimpering, infant-like being. The person will likely follow the doctor's orders, do the best to rehabilitate self, and likely, have minimal or no residual handicap. Conversely, the immature, hostile, impossible-to-please person squeals the loudest, often bringing about the most attention and accommodation. Yet, not only does he/she become more demanding and frustrating to cope with, having even more outrageous requests, but also expects and demands unreasonable compensation for slight injury. Such people do not follow a physician's orders well, put very little or no effort into rehabilitation, and are more prone to get a poor treatment result with maximal residual handicap. This patient example is currently in the process of destroying our insurance industry.

BLAME

Blame is an irrational phenomenon. Imagine a person using a hammer missing the nail and hitting the thumb. Someone is standing nearby. "Look what you made me do!" the person yells, an obviously irrational reaction.

Often the response is a very indignant, "I didn't make you do that!" Which is equally irrational. If the accusation is not true, no need exists to become defensive. Another inappropriate response might be a meek, "I'm sorry," which is also irrational, since nothing occurred about which to apologize. A rational response would be, "Gee, I bet that hurt."

Now we all project blame and we will until we die. This is one of the irrational aspects of being human. We are irrational, as well as rational beings, no matter how much we fight the idea. We are everything we have ever been, and the infant within us blames mother for everything for all time. When we were an infant this was a reality. Without her or a substitute, we die. The more threatened we feel—from within or without—the more prone we are to regression. Anyone near can become a mother substitute, and be blamed, be it spouse, parent, boss, child, or bystander.

Many people who come to my office initially state angrily, "Everyone in my family is blaming me and it is not my fault." They have, of course, never learned to listen to what the messages convey from the person speaking. They only look to the messages to tell them who they are and whether or not they have value. No one really has the right to tell us who we are and whether or not we have worth, even if they could.

Fortunately, blaming need not get us into trouble. It only does so, causing confusion or chaos and blocking communication, to the extent that we treat it as though it explains the reality. The most immature person is either never to blame for anything, or is always to blame for everything. The more mature person looks for a phenomenological understanding without resorting to fairy tales with monsters, victims, or rescuers. Unfortunately, too many of us spend our entire lives viewing people as monsters, victims, and heroes. The problem is everyone wants to be the hero, and if we are any one of the three, we are all three.

Many of my patients will spend a great deal of time and energy trying to convince me that they are complete victims, that they don't have a choice because..., and that they were made to do such and such. When the time is right for my response to be most useful, I respond, "What sort of knife or gun was used?" Great terror is involved in the realization that we are responsible for our choices, because it means realizing that we are without a parent or authority figure to take care of us in case one becomes necessary. The most immature patients will refuse even to listen to any suggestion that they are responsible for their behavior. For example, they are adamantly resistant to the idea that being late for an appointment was within their control. They are always victims of circumstances.

OVERPROTECTIVENESS

The overprotective person feels responsible for and has the need to take care of everyone, as though people could not take care of themselves. This necessarily includes giving relief if anyone has physical or emotional discomfort. The overprotective individual takes great pride in this attitude, and feels it is what makes him/her a good person, thus giving a sense of value or self-worth.

In my opinion, just as is a kitten or a puppy unique, we are as precious and special as we can ever be the day we are born. The reason we don't feel value later is because of the defenses we build up. As we grow up we become overly excited by experiencing fully the special infant within us. It makes us nervous to be consciously aware of its presence.

Overprotective people hear only one message in complaints from their children, spouses, or friends: "You are not a good person (or spouse, or parent) or else you would keep me comfortable like a baby, and I would not have any complaints or criticisms." Even such statements from a spouse as "You are not viewing me as being responsible for myself or capable of taking care of myself," are only heard as "You are bad."

Overprotective people are often so compliant, or helpful, that they provoke everyone around them. What frequently occurs is that they become very helpful and accommodating in order to try to achieve a desired closeness, while not comprehending that this very helpfulness ends up emotionally distancing (because it is insulting) the person desired. I say insulting, because it treats the other person as a weaker being.

A complicating deception in overprotectiveness is that the typical behavior to achieve closeness is simultaneously an unconscious subterfuge to prevent it. Overprotective people cannot tolerate intimacy. They initiate behavior and attitudes that are intended to gain merit for intimacy while protecting them against closeness. Sex is an obvious manifestation of closeness. Many patients complain of having no sexual desire for their mates. More frequently than not, the underlying reason is that they are not being honest with one another, in order to avoid conflict. They are being overprotective. The woman who pretends in order not to "hurt his ego" is insulting her husband. The man who performs or gives when he doesn't genuinely want to do so is treating his wife as though she is weak and threatening simultaneously. He thinks he does it because he cares, but he does it because he is afraid of disappointment and anger. He is also being overprotective.

Changed attitudes and behavior in this reaction pattern are very difficult to attain because the overprotective person must give up something that makes him/her feel very worthwhile (Poarch, 1987a).

NO

We can tell a great deal about people's level of maturity by their response to the word "No." In general, the more immature they are, the more they respond with outrage as though saying "No," were the same as beating a baby with a stick.

To say "No" to a very immature person or child is extremely hard to do because the reaction is so intense but if we try to avoid doing so the reaction may even be violent. If we fail to say "No," we become controlled by, or a victim of, the other's immaturity and, in effect are behaving in an equally immature fashion.

Although most pleasers consider themselves mature and see rebellious people as immature this is in fact not true. The more immature they are the more their desire to please blurs the reality and causes problems in saying "No." People do numerous things to avoid saying "No." They rationalize as to why the request should not be made, criticize with such terms as "selfish," "inconsiderate," or "immature" and complain about what a burden it is to be in such a position. The person or child making the request may even be treated as an enemy. To say "No" to a mature person is relatively easy because the response is more likely to be mild. At least it doesn't make one feel like a monster.

Many people cannot even say "No" to a door-to-door or telephone solicitor who is invading privacy without permission. How many people can say "No" to an invitation without an excuse? Many resort to downright falsehoods—irrational overprotectiveness. How seldom we say or hear "Thank you, I appreciate the invitation, but I'd rather not."

In a relative preference scale, most people want all births and no deaths. They want all hellos and no goodbyes and they want all "Yeses" and no "Nos." The extreme would be the person who will not attend funerals, will not visit someone in the hospital, does not learn to drive, never dates, and is still living with mother, "to take care of her," at age fifty.

GOODBYE

You can tell a lot by how a person says, or avoids saying, goodbye. Some people will never say it. They say, "See you later," or a similar phrase which indicates a reassurance. Other people will abruptly say, "Oops, gotta go," when there was no indication they were preparing to leave. This is a defense. If they must bear the pain of goodbye, which ultimately is the worst pain there is, they are going to get it over with quickly. This person in psychotherapy is prone to walk into a session and announce, "Well, this is my last session."

An example of trying to avoid the pain by delay would be friends who come for an evening visit. They will show up late. The appropriate time for them to leave would be about 10:00 p.m. They give no indication of leaving until 11:00, then mention it, but make no move. At 11:30 they stand up, but continue to talk. At 12:00 everyone is standing at the front door with it open. At 2:00 a.m. everyone, by this time quite exhausted, is still talking through the car window as it slowly pulls out of the driveway.

The examples are quite important. They represent extremes, but they symbolize the immense power of the effort to avoid the pain of goodbye.

Goodbye is a certainty. It is as inevitable as the death do us part phrase in a wedding ceremony. The more we fight it, the less freedom we have in living. Quite to the contrary, we live in fear of losing and the more we have to lose, the more fearful we become. This is why many people become more afraid and more symptomatic the more their dreams of marriage, children, career success, and economic success come true. The reason we are all so afraid of involvement, and the accompanying commitment, is because we know that the more genuinely close to another person we become, the more will be the pain of goodbye.

Patients will sometimes say, "I'm not going to continue to see you. I feel somehow you are going to hurt me." I respond with "You are right. To the extent we become involved we are going to hurt when we say goodbye. If that doesn't occur, you will have wasted your time and money here, so I hope the pain will be very intense for both of us."

Maturation is infinite. It is possible to continue to grow emotionally until we die. Unfortunately, many of us view emotional discomfort as abnormal, even as disease. Only good feelings are normal, we think. The idea, which is even embraced by many mental health professionals and physicians, is that emotional pain is quite separate from other types of feelings, and if unrelieved, will leave permanent scars, which collectively result in emotional problems. The problems are irreparable but compensable, resulting in a desire for other people and the world to repay them.

The reality is that growth is like learning to ride larger and larger roller coasters instead of trying to make life smooth and level like a freeway which soon becomes dull and boring. This growth-enhancing view is that emotional pain or distress, just as any other feeling, is something that will certainly change at any moment in time just as all feelings do. If we fight the feeling then it tends to hang on and fight back. The pain that we bear from our life's crises prepares us to cope with future crises and eventually our own aging, degeneration, and death. This is to say that growth can eventually make us able to accept and face our own mortality. The attitude that serves our best interest is that every crisis resulting in pain is an opportunity to grow.

AMBIGUITY

If our mother is very reliable and predictable at meeting our needs as an infant, we thrive. When she later begins to make us wait for her presence or for food, we are forced to face doubt and uncertainty. As we mature emotionally we must face progressively more ambiguity. To the extent that we do not learn to face ambiguity, we cannot become reliable and predictable enough to satisfy ourselves and others, and the world cannot be predictable enough to make us feel reasonably secure. As a result, we will then live in a more or less constant state of anxiety, fighting to control ourselves, others, and everything around us. We will resist all change, and since to adjust to change is necessary, we spend double energy by fighting it, and more energy to attain even a marginal adjustment. Immaturity/maturity then can be viewed in terms of a person's relative ability to tolerate doubt and uncertainty, more and more of which is required as we age and must face potential and real losses of friends and relatives.

In the extreme, people that cannot tolerate very much distress try their best to find a recipe or cookbook by which to live. They expect and even demand one of the psychiatrists. They try to be unreal or perfect which is the same as trying not to exist. Their grooming often makes them look like a clothed mannequin. Their house must be ready for a visitor at any moment: it must look unlived in, with everything in order at all times. In such interiors, one feels as if the floor should not be walked on, nor the chairs sat on. Change causes great distress and losses easily trigger a mood of doom. Ironically, the more answers this person gets, the more nervous they become and the more questions they ask. This goes on until the respondent becomes frustrated and refuses to answer, or says, "I don't know." They are only relieved by a response which makes it necessary for them to face ambiguity because the reverse only makes them request more and more certainty.

In short, by expending our energies in the direction of forcing ourselves to tolerate more emotional distress we grow in every way. If we spend our energies simply seeking pleasure and avoiding discomfort we will at least stagnate if not regress. The alarm in the pleasure center dooms us to defeat.

CHAPTER 3

THE DYNAMIC STRUGGLE

Emotional growth is a dynamic struggle. On the one hand are forces which try to produce sameness or comfort. In the extreme, these forces tend toward being overprotective, a term I described in the previous chapter. On the other hand are forces working toward growth, just as in flowers and trees. We all naturally seek that reaction that will foster our growth but we constantly test to see if the reactor is strong enough to be helpful. Any person or child seeking limits presents an example. Energy spent in the direction of growth generally leads to worry and guilt, exemplified by leaving our child with a baby sitter. Could any child grow emotionally if we simply avoided these feelings by not leaving? Our natural tendency is to avoid these painful feelings; therefore, much conscious effort is essential. Fear of risk or pain makes growth very difficult. It is the price we must pay.

Because of this dynamic struggle, every crisis we encounter throughout our lives holds the possibility of stagnation and regression, or growth and expansion. Fear can lead to helplessness, clinging and progressively more infantile behavior, or the opposite possibility, that is the opportunity to grow. If we face our crises, even though this results in great anguish, we discover our strengths and become less afraid of them. By this means we can discover that of which we are made.

You may now say, "But some people are simply stronger than others." I view all people as strong and weak as opposed to strong or weak. The main variable is the degree to which we are afraid of our weaknesses and how much we experience our strength as dangerous. Fear of one's weaknesses may result in defenses such as covering, denying or projecting them onto others. Men in our culture often project their fears, including fear of craziness, onto their wives. Many people, especially women, are relatively afraid of their strength. The latter often project their strength onto their husbands and feel quite vulnerable when he is absent.

The effort to cope with strength and weakness is rooted in the initial dynamics of emotional growth. Others have written about this struggle between risk and protection. Scott Peck's *The Road Less Traveled* (1978) is a good example to show the therapist's involvement in the process. Successful psychotherapists generally learn with time and experience that the more they worry without asking the patient for relief and the more they experience guilt because of being tough on a patient, the more the emotional growth, not only for the patient, but in like measure for the psychiatrist. The more they try to do things to reassure and relieve the patient of discomfort, which produces pleasurable feelings, the more they work against growth and, in fact, become destructive.

If psychiatrists are simply avoiding worry and feelings of guilt relating to their patients, they must necessarily be doing the same with their families. Extreme examples include giving tranquilizers to spouse and/or children and even performing electroshock therapy on family members. The psychiatrist is simply trying to relieve discomfort because he/she cannot tolerate sharing it.

The dynamic struggle between these two forces is occurring throughout our lives. *Overprotectiveness results in stagnation or regression. The absence of overprotection leads toward growth.* If we do not avoid emotional pain, we discover how well we can cope, which includes dealing with such immense losses as money, home, friends, parents, mates, and even our children. All of life's crises prepare us to cope with our own physical decline and inevitable mortality. As we are equipped to face and accept our mortality, we become free to enjoy living. Unfortunately, most people live their entire lives in fear of losing or trying to control sure losses. In whatever degree their behavior is determined by the fear of losing, they cannot enjoy the pleasure and benefits life has to offer.

INTIMACY

   MATURITY

      EMOTIONAL GROWTH

         LIMITS—FIRM YES/NO   vs.   OVERPROTECTIVENESS—LACK OF LIMITS

                         OVERSTIMULATION

                         IMMATURITY

                         BEHAVIORAL AND EMOTIONAL
                               PROBLEMS

Figure 3.1. Maturation Paradigm.

CHAPTER 4

STRESS

Contrary to popular myth, stress is not just a reaction to events in our everyday lives which causes us some degree of discomfort. **Stress** is related to *how much change we must adjust to in a given period of time.* Thus, positive events also cause stress. Examples are a much longed for first date, marriage, new home, promotion, or a great increase in income within a relatively short period of time. I have seen the latter result in alcoholism, accidents, illness, affairs and divorce. The positive or stimulating events make it much more difficult, sometimes impossible to maintain control of our impulses. Of course, the greatest stresses we must adjust to are birth and death. A new child in the family is a great delight, but all parents will agree it is also an enormous adjustment. When we have a loss, the more attached we are to that person or thing, the greater the wound. If we have a recent or current physical injury, for example, a fracture, then we will respond first to stress, even to changes in temperature, with increased discomfort in that area. The older we become, the more acute our awareness of this phenomenon.

No such thing as an unlimited tolerance for stress exists. If a soldier remains in front-line combat without relief, at some point he will become psychotic, get wounded, or both, if he isn't killed. All people are vulnerable, no matter what their hereditary makeup is or the number of great crises to which they previously have adjusted. Given too much change in too short a period of time, they may have an accident, or become physically or emotionally ill. Of course, more than one phenomenon can occur. I know of several instances where cancers were found soon after youngsters had gone off to college. A colleague had stomach cancer just after his father died.

Certain variables determine our ability to tolerate or adjust to stress. Of utmost importance is constitutional makeup, which is how we come equipped. Obvious examples of differences would be diseases or handicaps at birth, although we must remember some people even overcome great handicaps. Coping in spite of these may make them even more capable of adjustment than others. We are made of several systems, including skin, cardiovascular, respiratory, gastrointestinal, nervous, musculoskeletal, endocrine, and genitourinary. Not all systems have the same degree of strength or weakness. The weakest system tends to recur in families; that physical location where the family members usually respond first to severe stress, such as heart, lungs, skin, and intestines, all tends to be hereditary.

Central nervous system disease repeats itself in families. A more obvious hereditary disorder involving the latter system would be exemplified by Huntington's Chorea. The person develops muscular weakness progressing to paralysis, and eventually total involvement of the brain leading to dementia and death. Less clear in regard to heredity is a disease like multiple sclerosis. When an episode occurs, the severity of the period of weakness or temporary paralysis varies greatly in different people or in the same individual. In addition, the amount of stress required to trigger an episode varies greatly.

As we move in the spectrum from those that are more hereditary through those disorders that are in between, we come to those that are more clearly emotional. These include disorders where the limbic system or emotional brain and frontal cortex or thinking brain are involved. Some disorders that are more obviously related to the immaturity/maturity continuum, which are commonly referred to as the neuroses and personality disorders. These can be influenced greatly by treatment which fosters emotional growth and development.

Confusion reigns when we come to those problems referred to as schizophrenic disorders, which some professionals consider hereditary and incurable, and others consider a state of immaturity, or a temporary state of severe regression in response to stress. My view is that the problems that we commonly refer to as schizophrenic disorders represent a wide array of disorders and we should view schizophrenia as a symptom just as we do a fever, or hyperactivity in a child, with many possible causes. When the schizophrenic is in a severely psychotic state, we cannot know whether the extreme which the individual represents is due to heredity or immaturity, unless we apply treatment based on the growth and development model. We then can find out how much the person can be influenced to change and grow.

I have seen teenagers that would fit a diagnostic category of paranoid schizophrenia easily, who, fifteen to twenty years later, are extremely successful professionals. Some colleagues would say this history simply means the diagnosis was not accurate because paranoid schizophrenia is manageable, but not curable. Others would view it as I do: that paranoia, even to the point of psychosis, when treated simply as a problem with fear of aggression, it is quite treatable. Among the teenagers, one is now an attorney and another a college professor. However, I have encountered a few whom I have found impossible to impact significantly.

It is paramount that we not reify psychiatric diagnoses. The resulting ambiguity may be threatening, but it at least leaves our minds open. As long as the psychiatrist's and the psychologist's views are from the limited perspectives of normal and abnormal, sickness and health, we not only will continue to be burdened with trying to answer unanswerable questions, but also we will be looking from perspectives which are relatively primitive in terms of the development of psychiatry.

To summarize, stress is related to how much change we must adjust in a given period of time and we do not have unlimited tolerance for it. We begin with a certain constitutional makeup. Circumstances and events of life impinge upon that makeup, creating stress, with lesser amounts leading to minor symptoms, and greater degrees resulting in major symptoms. If we can increase our tolerance for stimulation and grow as described in the previous chapters, we can thereby change the threshold of our mental and physiological responses to stress. Then more stress is required before we develop symptoms of any kind.

SECTION II:

TRADITIONAL CLASSICS

CHAPTER 5

DEPENDENCY

Children have physical and economic dependency. All people experience emotional dependency. Even mental health professionals draw no distinction between the kinds of dependency. I believe the distinction is essential to any discussion of this topic.

An infant is obviously totally dependent on the mother or her substitute, else the child dies. If a mother performs tasks for a child who can perform those tasks for himself/herself, the child's continued growth and development is inhibited. Unfortunately, many mothers behave as if the child's brain will not let it, much less her, know if the child is hungry or needs sleep. Many treat older children as if their bodies can't distinguish temperature. They say, "Put your coat on. It's cold outside." The child has no choice but to fight if he/she has any chance of growing up. A mother behaving in this manner toward her child reflects her fear of the child being able to become independent of her. The mother who continues to mistrust her child's natural sense conveys to the child that his/her sense cannot be trusted. Subservient behavior will surely reflect the child's resultant mistrust in his/her own decisions, as though the mother were right all along.

I currently see a patient who becomes extremely anxious if she awakens during the night or does not get a certain amount of sleep. She also is overly concerned about what and when she eats because she has little trust in her natural senses.

Ideally, if we attain maturity, we no longer require anyone to meet our physical needs and we support our own economic needs. Thus, successful parenting results in our children not needing us physically or economically.

EMOTIONAL DEPENDENCY

A very useful procedure is to view emotional dependency as though we all have the same degree of need. Read on before you disagree. People need people, not more, not less, but to the same degree. The more we can accept this and *be unafraid to feel dependent*, the less we are afraid to be important to someone else or to have someone else be important to us, including our children. Obviously, these are equally interrelated.

We do vary as to how afraid we are of our dependency feelings. The outward **expression** or manifestation of extreme fear would be seen in people who feel they would die, or the only alternative would be suicide, if they lost their most significant dependency relationship. Now they experience this emotionally as the reality. The more they act as though it is the reality, and the more people around them react as though it is reality, the more irrational the relating. That is, the reactors reinforce the fear. Obviously, the fear does not come true because with only extremely rare exceptions, they survive, if the loss occurs. People have a tendency to view irrational people like this as more dependent or weak rather than just immature.

Now we turn to the **defense** against the fear of dependency *feelings*. We mistakenly think this is a better position, a position of strength. "I am very independent. I am strong. I do not need people. Everyone needs me." This person projects their dependency onto others and takes care of them, like a welfare worker might, in order to defend against, and vicariously meet their own dependency needs. It is essential for such a person to foster dependency in others. They rescue, loan money, bail people out, and endlessly polish their haloes for their behavior. This defense is very fragile and collapses if the person closest to them, usually the spouse, stops cooperating with the reaction pattern.

The resolution of dependency is to grow to enjoy feelings of dependency without experiencing the *feelings* as though they represent physical or economic dependency. Ideally, we feel more and more dependent on our long term relationships. We can only accept our dependency if we know that no matter how we *feel*, we could survive the loss of the one on whom we feel dependent.

The patients I see for long periods of time will *feel* more dependent on me, rather than less, with their improvement. This simply means they are less afraid of *all* feelings, which translates into more maturity. The more mature we become, the more we trust our intellect which tells us we can face separation, no matter how painful.

Summarily, the more mature, the less fear of impulses and more feelings of dependency. We can separate these from the reality which is physical and economic dependency.

CHAPTER **6**

AGGRESSION

The years of experience with behavior argue for the need of a framework or structure which parents, supervisors, and employers can use to set limits for themselves and their subordinates. Ideally, such a framework would make life more predictable and reliable for everyone. It also would be extremely useful to law enforcement officials and practitioners in the legal profession. Above all, its ultimate goal should be to promote emotional growth and development, thereby fostering better relationships, better functioning, and overall emotional health. This would result in a reduction of the frequency and severity of emotional problems. Such a framework touches and interacts with other sections of this book. I will approach it in terms of the fear of our own aggression. This includes the expressions of the fear and the defenses against the fear. Several variables are involved with a discussion of this framework. The first is aggression. I will then proceed to a discussion of the development of aggression.

I do not use the term aggression with a positive or negative connotation, but only as a term for something that exists in all of us. *Aggression is the initiative required to walk, speak, and make decisions.* I think it is a continuum between the simplest assertiveness, to irritability, to anger, then to rage.

I do not think people vary in regard to the existence of aggression: aggression is in everyone. In certain circumstances and at certain times, we can all kill. A mother may do so protecting her child. Men kill in combat. I view this potential as one's maximum aggression. *The variable then is not the aggression itself, but the fear of the aggression.* This fear is directly related to how much we trust our own ability to control our aggressive impulses, or how much we are *afraid* we are potential killers, rather than whether or not we can actually kill.

I think we are exactly, not more, not less, as afraid of our own aggression as we are the aggression of other people, although this is not apparent to most of us. This variable can be viewed as how much we experience our aggression as our best friend, of which we are the master, in the way a small child does when he says, "No! Me do!" That aggression makes us feel great inside, and not as though we are coming apart at the seams, or flying into a million pieces, as in a temper tantrum at the opposite end of the spectrum. The fear of our aggression manifests itself through such things as how cautious and careful we are, how deliberate, how much we are concerned about hurting someone's feelings, or making them angry, and even by the amount of tightness or hesitancy in our voice.

Dealing with the tantrum is going to be the model around which the framework for discipline is built, but first I am going to discuss some manifestations of fear of aggression. These exist in the form of **expressions** of the fear and **defenses** against the fear.

Some examples of expression would be the overcontrolling, dominating person who provokes people in order to test their resistance. If people show resistance, the person knows that his/her aggression is not that dangerous. The man beating his wife is behaviorally expressing his fear of his own aggression, actually wanting her to resist and not treat him as though he is dangerous. Characteristically, he is married to a woman who is afraid of being assertive and who constantly behaves as though he is dangerous, thus fostering the problem: a fifty-fifty deal.

Oppositional behavior, delinquency, and criminality are obvious examples of people wanting someone to stop them. They want to be reassured that they are not dangerous by having someone not be afraid of them. I believe people do not like or enjoy feeling dangerous and thus, by nature, are pushing people to stop them. Misbehaving children are actually very uncomfortable until someone stops them. Richard Speck, who killed several nursing students in Chicago, wrote with lipstick on a mirror, "Someone stop me!" Unfortunately, we have become such a permissive, overprotective society that the person who needs limits must eventually commit murder before we finally say, "Stop, you cannot do that."

Let us now look at some examples of defenses against the fear of aggression. These would include such things as shyness, passivity, obsessive-compulsive behavior, depression, and paranoia.

The *shy* child is expressing, "Don't be afraid of me, I wouldn't hurt you." Unfortunately most people respond by being very soft spoken and cautious with this child (as though he/she is indeed dangerous) and thus the shyness is reinforced. Conversely, if we are overly aggressive with the child, he/she becomes provoked, causing anxiety from fear of losing control, evoking inhibition, and more shyness. *Only if we treat this child just as we would any other child, will a reduction in the shyness occur.* Shyness then is a common way of holding back one's aggression in order to not take a chance on hurting someone or getting hurt.

Passivity is a defense in which a person defends against being aggressive by being unaware of anger, but behaves in such a manner as to provoke someone else to the extent that the other person expresses the anger for him/her. The other person does not realize he is doing this. Thus, the passive person may never become consciously aware of the anger, much less admit he/she has it, that is, owns it. The very innocent battered wife might be (but not necessarily) such a person. The husband who never participates in disciplining the children and allows his wife to make all decisions is another example. The wife whose problem complements his problems is constantly berating him and complaining about his passivity.

The **obsessive-compulsive defense** is very common in our culture. Many, if not most, successful people in business and the professions are relatively compulsive. They wear a straightjacket on their emotional lives in order to prevent the risk of being overly aggressive. Occasionally the seams split and they explode; then they feel miserable and start all over again trying to keep all aggression well contained. They commonly learn this defense from one or both parents. They may develop it as a reaction to parents who express the fear of aggression. Compulsives are frequently perceived as callous or uncaring because they remain so detached, even more so when emotions become intense (Poarch, 1987b).

Clear rules limiting doubt, uncertainty, and ambiguity are very important to obsessive-compulsive persons. Often they have a problem enjoying their success because the stimulation and power it brings makes them tighten up more. This leads to feeling more anxious and more deprived. (They are actually deprived of their own emotional life, but they feel it is their families and the people around them who are depriving them.) These people are usually careful and cautious and try very hard to please, to do things well, and they do not wish to cause feelings in anyone around them, especially anger. Feelings are to be avoided.

I would add here that any of these expressions or defenses can be mild or severe and different in degree from one day, one month, or one year to another depending on people's level of stress. The amount of change in their lives to which they are having to adjust at a moment in time is the determinant.

Depression occurs in people who experience their aggression as a monster within that must be kept chained else it will get loose and kill someone—namely the self. If they become murderously angry towards someone they love, they do not experience it as anger toward the person, child, lover, mate, or parent. They do not consciously realize it. Instead, they just experience suicidal feelings. The reader must realize that to experience murderous anger is not unusual. We all feel like killing our mothers millions of times while we are growing up, like the hungry baby does when she says it can wait a while on the bottle, or as the toddler feels when she leaves him with the baby-sitter.

In **paranoia** we also experience our aggression as a monster that must be chained for fear it will get loose and hurt someone, but this time for fear it will, at its peak, kill someone else. The paranoid person defends against losing control by projecting the anger onto the person toward whom the anger is directed. He/she feels the other person is the one who is angry. He/she may become convinced that the other person is going to harm him/her. Another complication is the fact that the paranoid person responds with rage toward any person who is spending energy and effort trying to help him/her. A very important point to remember is to not be solicitous when this person is being accusatory.

Fear of aggression manifests some of the developmental aspects of aggression. The infant's crying can be a way to exercise the child's heart and lungs or it can signal a need. If parents are overly alarmed at the cry and try in every way to prevent or stop the child's cry, then the baby can become the most powerful figure in the household. When this occurs, the person who is least equipped to administer authority has the most. The result is often chaos. Parents feel more helpless and exhausted and the infant more and more insecure and desperate. I have seen a mother so afraid to assert herself that she allowed her toddler to stand in her lap and pull her hair while exclaiming loudly to me that this was a sample of how crazy he was. I'm sure you won't be surprised when I tell you she was already divorced and that she conceived of her ex-husband as a monster.

Obviously, the child must come to feel that he/she has the power to signal needs and bring about a response, but if the child has more than that, the seeds of feeling dangerous are planted. The result is fear of aggression.

Not quite so apparent are the variables in the mother that determine the mother's response to the infant. The child can be aggressive at the nipple of the breast or the bottle when the milk is not flowing as rapidly as the child desires. The very timid mother, who will later not be able to discipline the child, may suffer quite an amount of pain because she cannot release the aggression necessary to pull away consistently and insist behaviorally that the baby be more patient. She may later tolerate the child's spitting and throwing food or dumping its plate, while she, as a martyr, presents spoonful after spoonful. This mother is defending against her fear of being aggressive.

Another mother may express her fear by pushing others to tell her to stop. She might have no patience with the infant. She may withhold food and basic needs at the slightest provocation. In the extreme she may slap or spank the infant far in advance of the child's being able to understand the meaning of the abuse. This infant may grow to be afraid to make a move or a decision for fear of being hit. I am here giving examples of extremes, but of course, all gradations are in between these.

The term *terrible twos* refers to a period when the child is trying to master his/her own aggression. We only refer to it this way because we do not know how to deal with it. To people who are not so afraid of aggression, it is not a terrible time. The child actually starts mastering some of his/her power with great feelings of pride when he/she does such tasks as drinking from a cup. Later, with being able to use spoons to eat and master more and more complex toys and influence parents with those feelings, there are greater and greater good feelings of oomph (strength) inside.

Gradually, usually during the twos, the child comes to say "No! Me do!" with intense determination. When the child *can do*, he/she feels great inside. If we do not allow the child to try, he/she is greatly dismayed and even this may cause such intense frustration as to bring about a tantrum. If the toddler is allowed to try and becomes increasingly frustrated because he/she cannot accomplish the task, eventually a tantrum will ensue which expresses the child's feeling totally out of control. This is a terrifying emotional state as can be seen in the child's face.

Most of us were reared by parents relatively afraid of aggression, but as parents we do the best we can with how we came equipped. Most frequently, we are equally as afraid of the child's inner terror as is the child. We respond by attacking the child, by spanking, just as was done to us. Translated, our behavior says, "I'll make you more afraid of me than you are of what's going on within you." Some of us will ignore the child, leave the room or even throw water on the child. Ideally we would pick the child up, hold the arms to the body with one arm and the legs together against our own body with the other. The child will squirm and cry with all his/her might to test to see if we can really maintain physical control and then, after a varying time, will relax. If the child was able to express words, he/she would say, "Gee, thanks! I thought that was the end of me." Our behavior is saying, "Ok, I will take over until you can regain control. Then you can start all over again trying to master your aggression and make more and more of it your best friend." The aggression feels like a best friend as long as one is its master, but the aggressive energy feels like one's worst enemy when experienced out of control and as expressed in a tantrum. A child has much difficulty in taking the risk of experimenting with increasing amounts of his/her aggression unless the child can depend on someone else to take over in case things get out of hand.

The older child who is excited because of a special guest coming to visit may behave as he/she would ordinarily never do. He/she might climb atop furniture or move frantically in a hyperactive state. Overstimulation has caused the child to lose control of behavior and he/she is not going to be able to enjoy the company, nor they the child's company, unless someone brings him/her under control, by saying something like, "Sit in that chair until you can regain control."

The same phenomenon happens before birthdays and holidays, especially Halloween and Christmas. This happens in toy stores. It explains why the stimulation of the sights and odors of the grocery store frequently make children very unruly and demanding to a very embarrassing degree if the parent is too inhibited to release the aggression necessary to discipline the child.

To summarize, just as with dependency in the previous chapter, the key is to distinguish aggressive feelings and impulses from the reality. This ability correlates with our tolerance for stimulation. We can have intense feelings of rage and violent fantasies or dreams without overwhelming anxiety. We trust in our controls and do not experience the feelings and impulses as indicators of behavior.

CHAPTER 7

SEX AND INTIMACY

Sexuality should be thought of in the same way in which we approached dependency and aggression; that is, in terms of fear, **expressions** of the fear and **defenses** against the fear. Expressions of the fear would include all the sexual deviations. Defenses against the fear might be exemplified by a person who is a prude, and a person who sublimates to deal with the fear, as a minister does. The latter's success, because of overstimulation, may cause his/her defense to break down. The scandals of the televangelism ministries of 1987 and 1988 illustrate the phenomenon. Rather than expand on the expression and defense approach, I choose here to take a different tack. Sex and intimacy are not separate issues, but the terms are not interchangeable because they do not have precisely the same meaning. Biologically, sex is the goal in relationships. Ideally, the ultimate positive expression of feeling between two heterosexuals, intimacy, would accompany sex. Unfortunately, this is the exception rather than the norm. The sex act can be no more than two people going through the motions to prove they can do it, such as experimenting young teens. Sex also may be much nearer mutual masturbation through use of another's body with the participants only adding to their autoerotic pleasure by doing it together. Sex can occur between homosexuals, who are not sexually differentiated and mature enough in tolerance for trust and closeness toward the opposite sex, so that they must settle for the limited pleasure of homosexual activity. Threatening as the thought may be to many, we all have the potential for homosexual activity. If this were not so, we could not love persons of the same sex. Homosexual activity is not an uncommon experimental activity at, or around, the age of puberty. Ideally, sex and maximal intimacy would be the same. Yet, if two ideally mature people were involved, sex and intimacy would not occur together in every instance because of the various stresses and strains in their lives. This is to say, the frequency and intensity of pleasure would still vary.

Intimacy is a continuum, beginning with simple attention and ending with sex as an expression of feeling. When we first meet someone, we often comment about a neutral topic such as the weather. If neither party is threatened, the conversation may progress to talk of increasingly more intimate topics like jobs, sports, spouses, children, backgrounds, and eventually to feelings or even dreams, although rarely at the same meeting. In contrast to conversation, the activities will progress usually from occupation or parenting activities in common, such as PTA or car pooling, to movies; observing sports; playing together at cards, golf, or tennis; then eventually to meals together; and possibly to sex. Sharing oral pleasures is next to sex for most of us. Obviously, this is oversimplified, but the process of conversation and progress of activities follow the pattern.

The desire for intimacy is not a variable, although it may not be conscious. The variable is our fear or how threatening our becoming close to another is. Attention is to intimacy as crumbs are to food. Some people can only tolerate attention, in which case they are like a person who could only eat crumbs of food because they are sure a whole bite at once would poison them. Entertainers commonly have this problem. Regardless of the amount of crumbs (applause) they may feel deprived and remain afraid of starving.

The principle variable which I feel exactly correlates with our ability to tolerate closeness without being overstimulated or threatened is our fear of being hurt or betrayed. In the extreme we may want a guarantee before we take a risk. This is exemplified in young teens when they are interested in someone of the opposite sex and they ask a friend of that person "Does she/he like me?" The hurt of which we are all afraid is losing that person with whom we allow ourselves to become involved. This ultimate betrayal is an absolute certainty even if it be death do us part. Lesser betrayals such as the person loving someone else, fantasized or actual affairs, are not the ultimate, although many people out of rage think, and even say that they would prefer the ultimate. Only to the extent that we can let ourselves be vulnerable to and accept the ultimate pain, in spite of our fear, can we tolerate maximal intimacy. In sex this would allow us to spontaneously and complete abandon ourselves, letting go of such things as judging and observing our actions, while in the act, or thinking about the act.

An example of fear of closeness occurs when a married couple achieves sexual intimacy on Saturday night. The degree of pleasure is maximal for the pair resulting in overstimulation. On Sunday morning husband awakens and makes an approach but his wife is not interested. He then becomes petulant and later demanding. This is certain to turn her off rather than stimulate her desire. He is soon accusing her of sexual frigidity. Fury mounts. She becomes apologetic and depressed. They consult a therapist the following week because of her sexual problem. His reaction to overstimulation was to regress to a complaining, demanding child. Her reaction was to become an overprotective mother and assume all responsibility. They are now distanced and no longer vulnerable to the dangerous overstimulation. Months may pass before Saturday's degree of intimacy reoccurs.

A husband commonly never realizes when his wife makes a sexual approach. He is so programmed to the idea that a man is always ready that he provokes an argument without even knowing why. In a therapist's office he may well complain, "She is never interested!" A woman may complain that her husband seldom shows any affection while she behaves in such an overprotective accommodating fashion that for him to feel intimate would cause him incestuous anxiety (Poarch, 1987a). If he is at all attentive, she begins picking up after him even more than usual, giving him helpful reminders and in general is especially attentive to his wishes just as a mother caring for an infant.

Many people mistakenly think that they could tolerate more passion during an affair because it was, or is, more exciting; that is they could let go to a greater extent. This is because the involvement is more superficial, and therefore, they have less to lose, which reduces the risk or pain.

Put in a different way, the desire is just like the air we breathe. All that must occur for us to become interested, progressing to care and concern, then to love, (to the degree of our tolerance) is for the other person to expose themselves not just in words, but in genuine, unstaged feelings. The person who can be emotionally revealing and is not afraid of intimacy will not feel deprived of it. The person who is afraid of intimacy will feel deprived and will tend toward blaming other people, such as spouse or parent for depriving them. This might be exemplified by a person you meet who talks for some time, but with no genuine feeling, and you don't remember their name upon next encounter. The opposite would be meeting someone who cried, and your heart went out to them immediately, and you automatically always remember them.

I have people come into a session and talk but it might as well be the desk or chair talking. No exposure occurs. Emotionally they remain detached. Obviously this is the problem that has brought them to see me. Often many sessions occur before I begin to be spontaneously interested and caring. This is a manifestation of their changing and growing. If I should try to convince them that I care before I feel it, they will not trust me, and appropriately so.

WOMEN WITHOUT DESIRE

Not uncommonly will a woman come to see me complaining of no sexual desire, or because her husband is complaining that she is never interested in sex. I first recommend that she never agree to sex unless she has desire. She responds by saying that she is not sure she would ever have any. I tell her that if she is to ever know, she must follow my recommendation. This most frequently brings her husband in to see me because he says that he has waited for periods of even months before and she has not shown any desire. I stay with my recommendation since nature is in my favor. More frequently than not, when she begins to acknowledge her own sexual desire rather than viewing it as only existing in her husband, he loses interest. Indeed, he sometimes becomes partially or completely impotent. Thus the sexual problem then was simply a manifestation of fear of closeness. It was a fifty-fifty deal, but out of her overprotectiveness she owned the entire responsibility for the problem as did the wife in a previous example.

WE RELATE THE SAME
SEXUALLY AS SOCIALLY

We relate the same way non-sexually as we do sexually, obviously, although that fact is quite surprising to many people. Some rather extreme examples, and others that are slightly less so underscore the reality. The examples occur in relative degrees and are not fixed. For example, men vary in degrees of impotence and the same man does not have the same degree of impotence at all times. The same thing is true for shyness, pain on intercourse, and other symptoms or traits.

A man who has never at any time in his life been sexually potent may meet you with a moist palmed, limp handshake, and flushed cheeks. He may have a scarcely audible to very soft voice. He may speak haltingly or in a mumble. I saw a college professor many years ago who was like this. His recurring dream was of pulling a string from his mouth without ever being able to get to the end. The string, of course, symbolized the umbilical cord. He had never been able to separate emotionally from his mother, and hence could not become involved enough for sex with another person.

Another example might be a woman who invokes in you immediately a feeling of tension. As you attempt to engage her in social intercourse, the tension doesn't decrease as ordinarily occurs, but continues to mount to the point of physical pain in some area of your body. This occurs because of the process of empathy or empathic communication. As a psychiatrist, I will not be surprised to learn that her main complaint is pain during intercourse, because I have already experienced it through the phenomenon of empathy.

The obsessive man, whose feelings are defended against by detachment and isolation of the feelings from consciousness, will often complain of a lack of responsiveness on the part of his mate. Less frequently he will complain of not being able to genuinely give away to passion and not experiencing much pleasure during sex with his partner. When he is talking he may communicate such lack of feeling that one is not moved to respond beyond a minimum, and may even be bored though the topic may be one that is ordinarily stimulating. Guffaw-producing jokes, when told by someone else, often fall flat when he attempts them.

This compulsive man is often married to a passive unresponsive woman, or an unreal, theatrical type. He would find others such as those in his imagination overstimulating, thus threatening his fear of losing control of his impulses. (This would cause him to find a way to drive them away long before marriage.) The unreal, unresponsive woman might well complain of lack of affection from her husband and a lack of desire for sex on her part. The passivity of one woman or the phoniness of the stagy one certainly is more likely to turn you off rather than on during social intercourse. The passive woman would be a flat respondent to jokes and the dramatic one would exaggerate laughs giving the spokesman no pleasure. Neither woman could tolerate marriage to the man she might fantasize because that would be overstimulation and provoke excess anxiety.

Another example is a man who, on first meeting, is so open and winning that you find him unusually pleasant. But as soon as you are won, that is you find yourself *emotionally* warming to him, the feelings suddenly dissipate and remain so. On consulting a psychiatrist he will complain of premature ejaculation.

Numerous more subtle examples could be listed, these communicate the concept that we all relate in the same manner sexually as we do socially.

Our patterns are consistent, even the way we relate to the clock reflects our pattern, but I will elaborate on this under the heading of "Time" in a different chapter. These examples convey how preposterous it is to think of sex as a separate and distinct area which is removed from relating outside the bedroom. I think that only out of threat or immaturity do people think of sex as if it were some bodily or physical function in a compartment removed from non-sexual life.

Parents frequently worry about the development of their child's sexual identity. If they set limits and impose consequences as recommended in this book, the child will relate well and the development of sexual identity need not cause concern.

To summarize, the dividends for risking the disappointment of "No" are seldom more evident than in the area of sex. Only by allowing ourselves to be vulnerable can we have any chance for involvement, intimacy, and sex. Redundantly, the greater our tolerance for pain the better our chances for gratification.

SECTION III

SETTING LIMITS

CHAPTER 8

TIME

Any discussion of limits must first and foremost deal with the issue of time. I view the measurement of time as a product of man. I do not think it can be wasted or saved, nor that one person's time is more important than another's, no matter how much he or she or many others may think so, even if the person is a physician with a full waiting room. An example of the very important person would include the football fan in Oklahoma who is too busy to have time, night or day, to do anything else, but with rare exceptions, always finds time to get to the University of Oklahoma football games. I think time was developed in order to arrange things for our mutual convenience. When primitive people were solely responsible for their own needs prior to cooperation, then they needed only to be concerned with the timing of seasons, plants, and animals.

I like to use time as a reflection of patterns because it is the fundamental equalizer. Since we cannot know when we are going to die unless we chose to control it by suicide, time is the one sphere in which we are all equal. We all relate in a very consistent pattern, even if it is a predictably unpredictable pattern, such as impulsive behavior. This is reflected in the manner in which we relate to our own inner-self (emotional life), spouse, children, friends, teacher, employer or supervisor, institutions, such as religion, government, law enforcement, and to the clock.

Those people who are always late, saying, "The clock will never control my life," also are relatively resistant, even rebellious, toward other people's expectations, wishes, and demands to the same degree that they react to the clock. The degree of resistance reflects the same degree of their immaturity, and they indeed are controlled by the clock although the control is negative control. They do not realize they are still controlled by it just as much as a rebellious child is negatively controlled by his/her parents! The decisions are not independent of the parent's decisions since they are still caused by the parents.

The opposite is exemplified by people who are always early and respond to the clock as though it is a matter of life and death. These people get progressively more panicky if any chance of being tardy exists. They cannot tolerate much discomfort within and cannot share the discomfort of others. They are always reassuring and tend to respond to discomforts, wishes, expectations, and frustration of others as though those are demands that they feel compelled to remedy. These actions signal a great degree of overprotectiveness.

BEHAVIORAL COMMUNICATION

If someone has an appointment with you, and that person is late, and you do not say or do anything, you are behaving as though they are more important than you. At the same time you are communicating non-verbally that you are afraid of them and that they are dangerous.

More often than not you wish to say something but you hold it back to avoid conflict. If you are late, you are communicating in behavior that you are more important, while testing the other person at the same time to see if they will respond as though you are dangerous, unconsciously hoping they will not. No one genuinely enjoys feeling dangerous or having others afraid of him/her.

The reasonably mature person, who views others as equals, can perceive of the clock as only a tool which is used to order things for our mutual convenience to make life more enjoyable for everyone. This person will be able to enjoy relationships with other people and not be still working out leftover childhood problems by treating others as though they were controlling parents, who must be fought, or as critical parents who must be pleased.

I have learned over the years that if I cannot find a way to get a patient to be on time, I cannot help him/her. At times this goes so far with chronic tardiness that I insist on the person agreeing to a contract that if he or she is one minute late, by my clock, I will not see him/her but the person must pay for the session. Obviously, I must be very careful to keep my clock with the radio time. This has only been necessary with a few patients. They always are one or two minutes late at least once just to test me, but so far, it has always worked to stop the tardiness.

Conversely, some patients are always early, but after a particularly exciting, overstimulating, session they, to their own disbelief, forget the next session. They are, of course, appropriately dismayed when I charge them. They say, "I have always been so good." Of course, if I do not charge them, they will never get close to that level of excitement again, and hence, I will be unable to help them grow beyond this point.

With regard to time, physicians and their patients are in a bind. Ideally, the doctor would stagger the appointments and both would be reasonably on time. Physicians often become more unreliable about time as they become overstimulated by their professional success. Commonly, their waiting rooms are filled. Out of the insecurity that goes with the doctor's responsibility, he/she has a tendency to view self as more important (or more godly) than other people to reassure himself or herself. To the extent that the doctor's patients and/or spouse let him/her get by with this, it increases the doctor's insecurity since he/she at least unconsciously knows very well that he/she is really just another ordinary person and can never be anything else. (I think we are all as precious and special as we can ever be the day we are born.)

Even though quite angry, patients add to the dilemma and tolerate the doctor's behavior because, in part, they also want to think of the doctor as closer to a god. Who wants to put their health in the hands of another mere human? Isn't this a bind?

The anger that we provoke when tardy or that we feel when someone else is late is frequently denied by all of us. If you think about how it feels for someone to treat you as an inferior, or lesser being, then you may easily realize the outrage that is denied.

If a person remains afraid of the clock or fights the clock, he/she cannot be an effective limit setter and disciplinarian. A very essential point is that one must overcome this resistance if one is to become able to deal with subordinates as a supervisor, or employer, or deal with children as a parent.

After editing this chapter, Gladys Lewis, whose husband happens to be a physician, wrote me the following note. I decided I needn't say more:

> You have raised a matter of great importance in health care. It is a source of immense frustration to people. I have changed ophthalmologists, gynecologists, and orthopedists during the past two to three years because I will not tolerate being entered into a fifteen minute time-slot with three to five other people. My seventy-nine year-old mother sat in an ophthalmologist's office two and one-half hours last week. The doctor was there all the time. It is an obscenity. I have never heard a professional address this. I hope you will extend this a bit farther to include the anger which ensues when we violate each other's clocks in our contracts. The same is true with any group or person who does that, but doctors are dealing with time and bodies. How much more personal can the rejection, albeit implied, be?

In summary the more we experience urgency in fear of time or fight the clock the more immature we are. Ironically these opposites are often married to one another. Only with maturity resulting from increased tolerance for stimulation can we react to the clock as a tool for our equal convenience which makes life more enjoyable.

CHAPTER 9

LIMITS

Most parents discipline out of their own fear, in an overprotective manner. When doing so, they are very sure of themselves but often end up treating the child as though its brain cannot be trusted with regard to eating, sleeping, or body temperature. A mother says, "You need a nap!" instead of admitting to herself that she is in need of some privacy and wants to be alone for a while. "Eat your food! You are going to get sick!" or "Put your coat on. It's cold outside! You will catch pneumonia!" are common statements that reflect a mother's mistrust of the child's brain. If she does this enough, the child will come to behave just as though she is correct.

The empathic communication between parent and child is very sensitive and accurate. We do not change our tolerance for pain quickly. Thus changing dramatically the degree of consequences we administer is a gradual process. By doing so we increase our tolerance for stimulation in both the pain center and the pleasure center. It takes months to years. Parents seeing me once per week for sometimes years fight change. They try to avoid the discomfort. Each wants the other parent to do what is necessary. "I do not want to be the heavy. My child might not love me anymore." In the case of a teenager, "He may run away from home," or even worse, "Deep inside, I'm afraid she might kill herself and I couldn't live with that." These are each different ways of saying I am afraid of my child in the latter examples, and I am afraid to grow up and be the parent in the first example.

Implementing the system involves growth and change. It involves increasing one's tolerance for frustration and emotional pain. It involves allowing one's child to be frustrated or unhappy without providing relief. We do not like for our children to be unhappy because we must share their discomfort. When they are emotionally uncomfortable, we are also. Not more or less, but equally. I want the reader to know that even if I am successful in conveying my ideas to you about limits and discipline and you thoroughly understand, it does not mean that you will be able to do it immediately, indeed, if ever.

I have come across many extreme examples during my years of practice. One mother told me that she was not overprotective because she was so less protective than her own mother. She informed me that her mother was famous for roping off the street during her naptime. This woman's husband was also overprotective as reflected by getting out of bed at two or three in the morning at his teenage daughter's request to prepare her a milkshake. The daughter's serious drug abuse problem was the manifestation of resulting lack of tolerance for stimulation.

Overprotective parents try so hard they are frequently outraged at the very hint that their behavior and numerous overprotective rules are not only not helpful, but even destructive to their child's growth and development. Currently, I am seeing a teenage girl's mother who had no less than five different mothers call her because they each wanted to be sure she knew that her daughter was not eating lunch at school. This daughter is an excellent student and athlete and also relates well to people. She does not avoid eating at home, yet all these mothers are afraid she might be anorexic.

The framework I am going to outline requires that we set limits firmly and back them up with clear, definite consequences. The limits are set to serve the child's needs, not to be protective. This requires a few rules. The only purpose of rules is to give the child a clear way of informing us by behavior if he/she is having trouble with controls and requires our help. When we respond with consequences, we may feel terrible at the time, but the dividends that come later will confirm that we have not been the villain, but indeed have been an effective, responsible parent. If parents' goal is to get to a point where they can avoid the task of saying "No" and administering consequences, they never will achieve it. If the goal is to get to where they are ready and willing to do the job if the need arises, the need will arise more infrequently.

Children only require this help when they are overstimulated or are anticipating overstimulation. The idea is to allow them to be otherwise free to experiment with more and more freedom. They can only do this if they know they can depend on us to step in and help out if they are losing control. If not, they must either become inhibited to the extreme of maximum withdrawal represented by psychosis, or they develop more and more serious behavior problems in expression of aggression.

We say "No" to a child to help him/her say "No" to self and others. As the children internalize more of the limits which we model, they can gradually increase the tolerance, or reset the alarms, in the pleasure and pain centers. Then progressively greater stimulation is required to cause loss of control. Of course, this is the process of maturation, which is the ultimate goal.

I shall now proceed to discuss examples of rules, overstimulation, and then consequences. Some overlapping will occur among these issues.

CHAPTER 10

RULES

Rules are the instruments used to set limits. Overprotective, immature parents often have far too many rules or none at all. Children need limits only to have a line to step over in case they need help with controls. Few are required but they must be clear. The rules are not for the purpose of protecting the child. They are not for the purpose of dominating in order to prove one's authority. Rules also are not for the purpose of hiding the parent's feelings of inadequacy.

We want our rules to foster the process of maturation. Parents provide rules to prepare the child for physical and economic independence. When successful, parenting results in an adult that is not physically nor economically dependent on another person, such as a friend or mate, unless by choice, as is the case when one parent chooses to remain home with the child instead of pursuing a career.

Maturation occurs as a person internalizes exterior limits and learns to formulate his/her own rules. When we allow children to ask again after they have been told *"No"* the first time, then we communicate that *"No"* doesn't mean *"No"*, but it means, "Ask me again." The child responds accordingly. Obviously a consequence should be present for asking a second time. The same consequence also should be if the child gets a "No" from one parent and then asks the other parent. If the second parent doesn't know the other parent has said "No," we nearly always find out later by coincidence. We then need to go back and impose a consequence *even if* the second parent also said *"No."*

I think the assumption can naturally be made that siblings will fight. I think they should receive consequences for fighting if the conflict is bothering the parent or if one or both children asks a parent to intervene by tattling. I recommend strongly that both children be punished equally. In this way, we simply make it pay for them to get along. After they are sensitized, then comments such as, "I can help you solve the argument," or "Do you want my help?" get an immediate response like, "No, we will work it out." In this way, we also get away from choosing "good guys" and "bad guys" or monsters and victims among our own children. The smaller or weaker ones soon learn to use this, or innocence, to their advantage if they discover we will intervene to protect them. We would have to be perfect or a god to be able to always choose who is right and who is wrong. My method not only reinforces siblings getting along, but it prepares them to relate in the adult world. If the earth were attacked from outer space, then no doubt nations at war would find a way to work together quickly. Parents must be the common foe, or the outer space attack, when their children are fighting.

After the "No" rules, we proceed with rules around time, since it is fundamental in learning to relate in the world. Bedtime rules come first. The more immature the parents, the more trouble they will have allowing an infant to cry even though the child has been fed, does not need the diaper changed, and does not have a fever. These same parents will have the most trouble making the child remain in bed when a toddler. Notice I did not say, "put to sleep," or "made to sleep." Obviously, we cannot make the child go to sleep, but we can insist it stay in bed. If the parents cannot find a way to accomplish this, then the child is more powerful than they. The person least equipped to administer power has the most. This increases the child's insecurity, and he/she has no choice but to keep pushing and testing in order to try to encourage the parents to prove they can take control. This is the only way it can feel more secure.

We want gradually to change the bedtime to a later hour until the child is nine or ten years-old, and then let him/her determine bedtime. We should then only require that he/she get up on time, regardless of when going to bed, with grave consequences if he/she does not. By this time, the child also should be using an alarm clock. Remember, if we do things that he/she can do without us, we are interfering with growth. The more the child does on his/her own, the greater the feeling of confidence and mastery. Giving up the task of awakening the child is sometimes very difficult. Parents I counsel often are amazed by the dramatic response when they stop.

Consequences must be great enough that to remain in bed is worthwhile for the small child and for the older child to give reasonable concern to getting to bed at a decent time. You may be questioning, "What are some consequences?" This is the most frequently asked question in my office. I assure you we always are able to come up with some. I can tell you with reasonable certainty that *if your motivation is protective or the consequences not great enough, the child will not relax and will continue to press the limits.*

Parents may discipline their child for being in a *bad mood, for talking back or for using foul language.* I disagree with all of these. Although each example is usually an expression of overstimulation, they are just words, not weapons. When these things are occurring, *behaviors,* such as rule breaking or lack of carrying out ordinary responsibilities, have already occurred and are being overlooked or ignored. Some examples might be a forgotten chore, the room not straightened, or some kind of tardiness. Discipline should ideally only be for behaviors resulting from overstimulation, which is causing the child to lose control of impulses, not for feelings, moods, or verbal expression. Amazingly, *children ask for help with self-control by misbehaving.* They change dramatically in mood and verbal expressions and again become pleasant company when we give appropriate discipline.

As already established in the chapter on aggression, when the child can trust that we will take over when help is needed, then he/she will experiment with more freedom and more stimulation to see how much can be tolerated without losing control. This will result in a progressive resetting of the alarm in the pleasure center of the brain. When we provide consequences which are severe enough in controlling the overstimulated child, this modifies the excitement.

Progressively more severe consequences increase the tolerance for pain in the brain's pain center. As parents, when we do provide such consequences, we increase our own tolerance by the same degree. We grow also. This results in *what is genuinely good for one being equally good for the other.* Obviously, this overcomes the idea of "good guys" and "bad guys," which is a product of *fairy tale thinking.* Fairy tale thinking refers to ideas about people which are the residual of the oedipal romance of childhood. Most fairy tales are the symbolic expression of this romance. When we divide people into monsters, victims, and rescuers, it makes things very simple. We all then want to be rescuers or heroes, but the problem is we cannot be one without being all three. This system of thought also requires that other people be monsters and victims.

ALLOWANCES AND MONEY

The second main area regarding limits is money. If one is going to be able to relate reasonably well in the adult culture, an essential component is that one be able to live within the constraints of time and money. The better our preparation as children, the better we will be able to adjust to these limits as adults. Obviously, those children who are not required to carry out any responsibilities in order to get an allowance and are given money upon request are at a disadvantage as adults. They expect to have all of the pleasures and privileges which money buys. At the same time, they are outraged at the thought of having to earn it. Far too many adults have had such rearing which results in the self-defeating abuse of credit cards, failure to pay regular bills, overspending at Christmas, and at worst, bankruptcy.

An opposite problem are those adults who think of money as a way of keeping score in regard to their adequacy or success. This can lead to unnecessary pressure and an impractical view of money. We can also prevent such problems by the way in which we treat our children in relation to money.

Children who have been required to earn and save money, and who could not buy the larger or special items when they did not have the money, are much more realistically prepared for adulthood. Those who have been indulged often become adults who expect to receive or get a great deal with little effort, and they end up spending a great deal more money than their income. Unconsciously, they work harder and harder to get rid of whatever money they have. By nature, they are trying to get rid of their money so they will be required to face reality and grow up. Unfortunately, too frequently they are rescued by well meaning friends and relatives.

Often learning about money begins when toddlers ask for candy or gum in the grocery store. I will elaborate on this issue in the chapter on overstimulation. An important procedure is to begin giving them an allowance at a very early age. This should be increased progressively as they grow older. Also the allowance needs to be given on time. As an adult, we are not required to ask for our paycheck, and children should not have to ask for their allowance. Children should have one or more chores they are required to perform in order to get their, allowance. If the task is forgotten, not done promptly, thoroughly, or without reminder, they are to be fined a substantial portion, if not all of the allowance. An effective way to promote savings is to require that a percentage of the allowance be saved under penalty of loss of all the allowance. An alternative is matching savings as an incentive, but if this is overstimulating, the child will save less, not more. Such a plan teaches the importance of saving, a desired lifetime habit.

Many parents complain that their children do not think about getting cards or gifts for family birthdays, or even Christmas. Small children will often spontaneously make gifts for siblings or parents. If we do not treat children like they should not have to worry about having to make or find gifts, they will also spontaneously begin to use their savings to buy birthday and Christmas gifts for siblings and parents. The important point is that they be able to use their allowance and savings, and not be given extra money or have gifts bought by parents for them to present. The latter promotes immaturity and irresponsibility.

As children grow older, they need to open a savings account at the bank. As they accumulate money, they can deposit it into the savings account. Now I do not mean that the parents should open the savings account for the child. I mean that parents should take the child to the bank and let the child open their own savings account. Later, during the mid-teens to upper-teens, youngsters need to have a checking account. This teaches the child more and more about our monetary system and does not leave them naive about banking.

Some children even buy stock or Krugerands with their savings, and thus learn to invest during their teens. Some youngsters start with a paper route and buy special bicycles of their own. Some save money for a portion, if not all, of a car as they get older and get increasingly better jobs. This system also motivates them to obtain part-time jobs and summer employment at an early age.

For parents, their youngster's ownership of a car is an enormously significant issue because so many teens are injured or killed in auto accidents. My opinion is that the more youngsters pay out of their own earnings and savings to buy their own car, the less likely they are to get speeding tickets, injuries, or end up dead as the result of an accident. Obviously, a helpful procedure is for them to earn the money to maintain the car and to pay the insurance. When a youngster earns the money for his/her car, the tendency is to take much better care of that car. For parents who can easily afford to pay, it becomes very difficult for them to slap their own hands. We enjoy giving. To resist and require more of the youngster is much harder to do but far more caring.

TELEPHONE

To communicate in writing is very safe as exemplified by children passing notes. This is because the response is not immediate. Next most safe is talking by telephone because no touching or hitting can occur. Teenagers love to talk on the phone as they are gradually risking greater involvement, especially with the opposite sex. They may easily get sidetracked with this level of relating and not risk the less safe face-to-face relating.

We can help by setting some limits. Unless an emergency occurs, youngsters should not be allowed to receive or make calls after ten o'clock in the evening. Also a time limit should be established per call such as ten to fifteen minutes. If abuse occurs such as overtime or calling again a few minutes later, phone privileges should be withdrawn for several days. Parents need not worry about constant monitoring. If the youngster is abusing telephone privileges and parents are unaware, the youngster will make the deviate behavior more obvious in order to seek help with restraint.

In summary living with clear rules allows us to know when our controls are breaking down and we can begin trying to ascertain what is going on in our lives which is overstimulating. Clear rules for our children or any subject in an authority-subordinant relationship allows the authority to know when help is needed.

CHAPTER **11**

OVERSTIMULATION

Overstimulation is that point at which pleasurable or painful stimuli, relative to a person's or child's conditioned tolerance, causes anxiety for fear of losing control, and if the stimuli continue unabated, the loss of control. Take the example of a small child accompanying a mother to the grocery store. Obviously, the odors and colors are overstimulating and it is naive not to expect that the child will wish for many different things, such as candy and gum. An unruly, unreasonable child is nearly impossible to deal with in the grocery store. The scenario is a very common one. Preparation for the experience can be made by setting a clear limit of some kind prior to going to the store, such as "You may have one thing, but it cannot cost more than twenty-five cents." This is a clear limit. Telling the child it must behave is too broad. The manageable limit is also going to be useful to the child in learning the price of items, because the questions, "How much does this cost?" will be necessary in making a choice. The limit also begins the initial education regarding the value of money. The child *must know* that it cannot go above the limit. Serious problems will follow if the parent bends, for example, saying, "Oh, well, okay, I guess so, that costs thirty cents, but I will let you have that." By this I mean, the child cannot trust the limit because it is not really firm.

The very act of setting a limit increases the odds of the child's being able to maintain control in spite of the intense stimulation in the grocery store. If the child cries and complains again and again to get around the limit, the parent must be willing to deal with the child, then and there. The parent must be able to say, "If you are going to give me a hard time, then you can't have anything." If that means promising the child that they are going to get a spanking when they get home, and that works, that is fine. If it requires spanking right there in the grocery store, then it must be done. If children sense that in public you are not going to deal with them because of being observed, then when they are stimulated they feel no sense of safety control from your presence and they become increasingly more insecure as they get more stimulated and you have a progressively greater problem. Even parents that are not afraid to deal with their child in private are often afraid of their child in public, and then the child's insecurity intensifies. Ironically, just when you are most wanting them to be well behaved will be just when they are most likely to become out of control and embarrass you.

Inhibited, shy, or constricted parents may well have children who are overstimulated very easily. Simple things such as mastery and success can cause the child to require discipline. We can get by with giving a child lots of stimulation if we are willing to give appropriate limits and consequences. Most people love to give to their children, but they hate with a passion to discipline. When a child is out of control, we can obviously do one of two things: we can reduce the stimulation, or we can add consequences. We may be required to do both.

Obviously, after children have spent some time at an amusement park, whether the amount of time there is one hour or until the gate closes, they are very likely going to be overstimulated and have a difficult time adjusting to the ordinary. Just when you think they would be most appreciative, they are complaining with a frenzy and are the most unpleasant company. Not until you institute some form of consequence will they settle down, perhaps cry, and then go to sleep in the car on the way home. If you avoid doing this, then everyone is going to have a very difficult time for hours or even days.

Grandparents and non-custodial divorced parents are frequently indulgent of children. After spending the weekend a child often returns home unruly or frantic. In fairy tales, grandparents are symbolized as fairy godparents. One of the advantages of being a grandparent is having the power to make children's dreams come true, then avoiding the task of dealing with the resulting overstimulation by sending the child home to parents. If, as parents, we avoid giving consequences immediately after we pick them up, or on the way home, then we can have problems for several days. This example frequently comes up in my office.

Obviously, a mother's excitement can be empathically picked up by the smaller child and cause it to have difficulty maintaining control. Conversely, a child's excitement and stimulation is picked up by the parents. We enjoy our children's excitement, but it sometimes creates difficulty for us in setting limits or instituting discipline because we are having trouble maintaining control ourselves. Nothing delights us so much as the excitement of our children as long as they are in control of themselves.

Prior to holidays, such as Halloween, birthdays, and Christmas, children are much more stimulated. Instead of concentrating so much of our energy on making happiness and enjoyment for the child to the extent we would desire, we must help the child with control when necessary. I have heard a child speak spontaneously responding to the mother who has just said, "Now we must be happy" with, "I don't want to be happy!" He was trying his best to make it clear to the mother that she was overstimulating, and it was making him miserable.

In school children, particularly older children, stimulating occasions include the time just prior to anticipated events: spring break; summer vacation; important occasions, such as school proms; very important dates; before as well as during vacation trips; and when anticipating or while spending the night with a friend. An especially stimulating time is when parents allow the child to take a friend along on a trip. Very likely the youngster is going to require more discipline at these times. Often parents feel that just when they are trying so hard to give the child pleasure, the child is least appreciative. The child is just insisting on some help with controls.

The big stimuli that make for grave danger are such things as motorcycles and cars. I frequently say that the child who screams the loudest for a motorcycle is the last one who should have one and the most likely to get himself/herself injured or killed on it. In general, such things as a cycle for a thirteen to sixteen year-old youngster are dramatically overstimulating, and the likelihood of a youngster that age being able to deal with that degree of stimulation is almost nil.

The recently outlawed three-wheel vehicles and off-the-road bikes that fathers and children often enjoy so much are quite dangerous and the excitement is so high that it is nearly impossible to institute enough discipline to help a child maintain control. Many parents who come to me with behavior problems in their children are eventually required to take away and dispose of these kinds of vehicles in order to help the child. Recently a family had to get rid of a Christmas go-cart because their twelve year-old's grades fell. With the consequence, his grades improved right away.

When parents are considering getting their child a car, just the anticipation of being able to drive is often overstimulating to the youngster. When we add to that the prospect of owning his/her own car, much less getting one as a gift, often the result is speeding tickets, and if the car is not taken away for a period of time as a consequence, then the chances of accidents are greatly increased. Paying the fine is not nearly enough.

BRIBES

An extremely important point to understand is that bribes nearly always result in the opposite of that which is consciously intended. As parents, we may unconsciously wish the child to fail so he/she will remain dependent and cannot become self-sufficient enough to do without us. When parents bribe their children to eat or to meet ordinary expectations, such as picking up after themselves, or making the bed, they are conveying to the children that they are less than adequate. Children will respond accordingly.

Success is its own reward and it is difficult enough to tolerate this stimulation. When we add the stimulation of a bribe on top of the excitement of the success, we decrease the likelihood of the child being able to succeed because they must fail in order to prevent the anxiety caused by overstimulation.

A teenage girl had always performed poorly in school and never near her ability. After her parents had begun instituting a program of limits and consequences, she was beginning to perform better and also to enjoy school for the first time. The father then offered her a new car if she would make straight "A's." Suddenly, instead of enjoying school, she was feeling a great deal of pressure regarding school work and it was making her miserable. Obviously, the pressure would reduce the likelihood of success rather than increase it.

A similar example is that of a colleague's patient, a teenage boy who, because of alcohol and drug abuse problems, was hospitalized. He had frequently been truant and performed very poorly when he had attended school. After discharge from the hospital, he soon was performing so well that his parents were overstimulated. They then presented him with a new car. The following week he failed to attend school and the next weekend received a traffic citation for driving under the influence of alcohol. When my colleague had the boy read some of my material, the youngster said, "Are you going to recommend they take away my car?"

DANGER

Parents puppy wrestling and playing horsey with children is great fun for all parties involved, but a common error is for parents to enjoy this kind of stimulation just prior to bed time and then expect the child to turn off immediately like a light bulb. My response to such expectations is "good luck."

One man, who had habitually wrestled with his daughters then ten and twelve years old, consulted me with intense anxiety after beginning to have partial or complete erections during the play. He was desperately afraid that he might be perverted. It was, of course, time for him to cease such activities with his daughters.

A child cannot maintain control for any reasonable period of time when parents insist on certain activities. These things include the mother continuing to sleep with her son that is four or five years old. At this stage of maturation, he is trying to master his romantic feelings. This is the age when children love the romantic fairy tales like "Cinderella" and "Hansel and Gretel," which are about the family romance (Poarch, 1987a). The child is going to have severe nightmares. He/she is also going to have a continuous behavior problem, and as long as the mother continues to let the child sleep with her, almost certainly the symptoms and behavior problems will continue in spite of discipline. This overstimulation is nearly impossible for the child to tolerate and if forced to try, up to and through puberty, the likelihood of severe symptoms such as psychosis are extremely high. I have seen an example of this in my own experience. A boy in his early teens had continued to sleep with his mother. He would get up to change the television channel and step forward and backward in one place for up to twenty minutes.

Ordinarily children block out the overstimulating images of their own parents having sex unless the behavior of the parents overcomes the child's defenses. Such behavior would be exemplified by nudity and sexual petting in the presence of the children. Psychic defenses are more difficult where step-parents and adoptive parents are involved. Since the incest taboo is not as strong, sexual images are more prone to find their way into the conscious awareness of the child. When a single parent allows a guest of the opposite sex to spend the night without making separate sleeping arrangements, children are going to be dramatically overstimulated making disciplinary efforts futile.

A child of about three sleeping with the parent, especially of the opposite sex, is sometimes so overstimulated that the child may experience a burning in the stomach. The child cannot express this except behaviorally. He/she may then begin playing with matches, become more and more interested in fire, and begin to light fires in order to express, "I am burning inside." Unless the stimulation is reduced, the fire setting will become more frequent and severe.

Preschool children naturally develop modesty regarding dressing and bathroom activities unless parents chide them. Bathing and showering with children above toddler age may be convenient to very pleasurable for the parent but is definitely overstimulating for the child. Such behavior is going to produce very inhibited or very unruly children. I recently saw a young father complaining about the obnoxious behavior of his four year old daughter. She changed "amazingly" when they stopped bathing together.

I also want to make it clear that no such thing as an unlimited tolerance for pleasure exists. People do not at some point become able to tolerate any amount of stimulation. Evidence of this would be exemplified by Gary Hart's indiscretions when it appeared he might have a good chance to become president of the United States. President Nixon's continued rule breaking led to the Watergate hearings when he was in his second term of office. This phenomenon could have been involved in the Iran-Contra Affair. A second term in office during peacetime is possibly too much power, thus overstimulating, for a mere human. Perhaps the second term in office during war-time cannot be interpreted as a personal mandate for a president, and so does not result in such overstimulation.

Other examples of adult overstimulation are those such as doubling a person's income within a short period, as has occurred sometimes in the careers of securities traders, real estate brokers and oil men. To tolerate or adjust to that much change in a short timespan is very difficult. The likelihood of the person developing marriage problems, even resulting in divorce, alcohol abuse, drug abuse, illness, or having an accident becomes much greater than it otherwise might be.

One prime example of dramatic overstimulation resulting in drug use would be the professional athlete, who fresh out of college, receives a huge sum of money. This makes him feel less pleasure rather than more, due to detachment from emotion to defend against the stimulation. Often the result is drug use and gambling. The drugs are used to overcome the alarm in the pleasure center so that he can feel alive again. The gambling is to get rid of the money so as to reduce the stimulation.

OVERSTIMULATION
IN THE PAIN CENTER

Section III of the book discusses, primarily, issues related to overload in the pleasure center of the brain. Obviously, overstimulation in the pain center occurs, but the questions arises, "Does it require discipline?" When the result is a chronic morose state or prolonged emotional withdrawal as seen in some teenagers and adults, but less frequently in children, it does not. These reactions occur after major losses or trauma and should be treated by experienced mental health professionals.

In children and younger adolescents the reaction is much more commonly manifested as a behavior problem. For example, a child who is ordinarily well behaved at school is quite unruly on Monday morning. His teacher asks him if something is the matter. He responds resistantly, "Nothing! Leave me alone." The teacher informs him that he will not be allowed to go outside for recess because of his rule breaking. He immediately breaks into heart-rendering sobs, quite out of proportion to the disciplinary measure, and after a few moments he reveals that his mother is in the hospital because of an injury sustained in an auto accident. His overstimulation was in the pain center and consequences for his lack of control provided relief, just as they do when the overstimulation is in the pleasure center.

Unfortunately, children who have had major trauma or losses are treated as though the events should not have happened. The result of this kind of overprotectiveness leads the children to believe they should not have to cope with such events. To cope with something is very difficult, if not impossible, if the people on whom you depend to help you test reality are giving you the impression that you should not be required to cope.

A child who has sustained the loss of his/her mother early in life may refuse to be involved with a foster parent or step-parent or to develop meaningful friendships. Hostility is the most common reaction to the efforts made to engage such a child. This state of affairs will persist until someone has the courage to be tough and consistently set limits and impose consequences for misbehavior. Sympathy often interferes. One child whose mother died when she was two years of age was brought to see me when she was nine. She was determined never to let anyone be close to her. Silently we played games for several years before we had anything that could be called conversation. It was very difficult to train her parents to be firm. She needed extreme toughness. Successful therapy required eight years of once-per-week sessions for her and her parents. Early in the process, while she was still resisting talking to me, her father asked her how long she thought she would continue seeing me. To his bewilderment she responded, "Until I am sixteen." Translated, this says, "When I am not afraid to grow up, as reflected by driving, I will no longer need Dr. Poarch." This is an example of the confirmation of the unconscious awareness of the process of growth.

I also had occasion to see a boy, age eight, who had, at the age of four, observed his father brutally murder his mother and seriously injure an older sibling. His father had remained in a mental hospital since the event and his several siblings had been placed in separate foster homes. Everyone who had significant contact with him was informed immediately of his past trauma. Of course, their emotional reaction was intense, and they responded to him just as though the event had occurred yesterday. No one reacted to him as an ordinary boy. How could he be expected to cope when virtually everyone, including his teachers, were treating him as though he was not whole.

Fortunately, most of us are seldom required to deal with children who have such extreme overstimulation in the pain center. I will close this subject with a statement I wish for all readers to remember. *To expect a child, indeed anyone, to trust a person who reacts to overt hostility or very unruly behavior with sympathy and kindness is preposterous.*

In this chapter I have presented evidence which makes it clear why I assert that forcing ourselves to tolerate more stimulation in the pleasure center is impossible. At that point when we become overstimulated our controls break down. We therefore "blow it" every time.

CHAPTER **12**

CONSEQUENCES

Virtually all parents seeking my consultation regarding limits and discipline begin by trying to convince me that they have tried everything. Whether the child we are talking about is a toddler who won't stay in bed, an eleven year-old who simply refuses to do homework and school assignments on time, if at all, or a teenager drinking and staying out late, we begin with an utterly impossible task as far as the parents are concerned. Each of these three instances must be individualized to certain extent, but I am going to share with you how we proceed with this task.

In the case of the toddler, I discovered that his young mother adopted two delightful children after having given up on having a child of her own. To her surprise *and* amazement, she then became pregnant. After this baby was born, she and her husband could hardly contain themselves, and were both having a very difficult time keeping their feet on the ground. Because of their overstimulation, their middle child, the toddler, was empathically sharing and expressing their excitement by finding it impossible to remain in bed. I then discovered the older child, age five, was uncharacteristically unruly, refusing to obey, and the mother was finding herself unable to let the new infant cry. She was always picking it up in spite of knowing she should be able to allow the crying. Thus, because of their excitement, the parents were finding it impossible to control any of their children.

In such a situation, the children will keep on testing and pushing, making life more difficult for the parents until the overstimulation of the parents is modified. The children will bring the parents back to earth. After I pointed out what was happening, the parents were no longer so bewildered and scared. Then they did not need to be convinced that they had the power to control the children.

The parents both had a history of inhibition and over control. This constriction was the manifestation of their relative lack of tolerance for stimulation. The latter causes a problem in ability to release the aggression necessary to control the children when needed. This example makes clear that problems in children do not occur independently of problems in parents.

In the instance of the eleven year-old, I found that the boy had a phone, television, and stereo in his room. He also had a motorized bicycle, played soccer, and his father was the coach of his team. His mother was overcontrolling, out of her own fear, and the father self-indulgent, which was made apparent by his being severely overweight. The boy was living like a millionaire, while performing in such a manner as to be fired from any employment, were he an adult.

My first task was to convince the parents to change the boy's life-style to fit his performance. School is the child's primary occupation, just as an adult's employment is the primary occupation. If the adult does not perform adequately, then immediate consequences will occur where one's life-style is concerned. When we allow children to perform at a level less than their ability, we are insulting them. Our behavior is saying "You are not adequate, therefore we cannot expect as much from you," or even, "There is something wrong with you; therefore, we cannot expect as much from you." These messages have a profound impact on all aspects of the child's life. For a child to be allowed to participate in any extracurricular activities, when he/she is performing at less than its academic ability, is preposterous.

The last thing the father of the eleven year-old wanted to do was eject his son from the soccer team because of grades. Also just as obvious is that what is the most difficult punishment for the parent to administer is also the most effective. The child unconsciously knows, without doubt, that such an act is performed only because the parents truly believe it is in his best interest.

In the upper teens, jobs to support luxuries are a frequent source of conflict between parent and youngster. Since outside work is a privilege, not a right, this means that the teen who was allowed to work while going to school would be required to quit the job if studies suffered. Of course, the youngster who really needs to work would probably not be suffering from overstimulation. Below ability grades are seldom a problem in the latter situation.

If reducing the source of the overstimulation is not enough, then we must add consequences, such as fines, grounding, no television, no phone, and more chores. In older teenagers, if grounding doesn't work, then we must move toward no recreational driving. By this, I mean driving only for parent's convenience. If this is abused, then no driving at all is permitted for one to six months. Sometimes we must become quite innovative with restraints. For instance, nothing worked to help a fifteen year-old girl, until I noticed that she was dressed in a different outfit each week when she came for her session. All of them were quite becoming. I suggested to her parents that they take away one outfit for each transgression of rules and return one only if no rules were broken for one week. Along with this, she was not allowed to borrow any clothes from her friends or her mother, which she had previously done. She became more pleasant company and her school performance improved.

I think all teenagers should have an agreed upon curfew. Youngsters should ideally have some input about their schedules, but if they do not participate reasonably, they give up the opportunity to share in forming rules. The time should be the same Sunday through Thursday, and later on Friday and Saturday during the school term. The hour can be changed for school functions and for special events if the change is discussed as early as possible. This fosters planning and responsibility. It might be appropriate to allow a small child to spend the night at the time he asks but not an older child. When we allow last minute changes or planning we treat the youngster like a three or four year-old and foster immaturity.

If a youngster comes in five minutes late and we do not impose a consequence, for example, grounding for a weekend, then we are saying, "I'm afraid of you," with our lack of response. A parental lecture or critical responses do not count. The five minutes late behavioral message is, "I'm having trouble handling my freedom right now because of overstimulation and I need your help with control." Predictably, the youngster will come in twenty to thirty minutes late after the next outing. If there is no consequence, or if the consequence is not severe enough, the youngster will then come in two or three hours late, and in the meantime be using alcohol or drugs to turn off the alarm in the pleasure center so that he/she can falsely enjoy the freedom. As you might imagine, by this time, the parent or parents are nagging, criticizing, guilting, and shaming the youngster, as well as themselves, while avoiding the task of dealing with the behavior. Real and severe enough behavioral consequences might include taking the car away, or even stripping the youngster's room to a bare minimum. Consequences are often deterred by the youngster's threats of running away or suicide, the likelihood of which becomes greater each time such threats decrease or influence the parents' decision to be firm. This becomes so because the parent's behavior is saying, "We are *afraid* of you. You are indeed dangerous, just as *you* are *afraid* you are."

Parents are our original reality testers. If an adolescent is already afraid he/she is dangerous and parental behavior reinforces this feeling, anxiety increases and the youngster has no choice but to keep testing and pushing. If parents fail to deal with continued tardiness, the most frequent result is the teenager's remaining out all night on several occasions and if the parents remain ineffectual, the youngster will run away. The young person is unconsciously seeking some authority substitute to respond behaviorally in such a way as to say "I'm not afraid to deal with you. You are not dangerous." This will eventually lead to contact with police. Unfortunately, at this point the adolescent often only receives more threats and lectures which are not helpful. These are just what caused the runaway. Obviously, the youngster's anxiety is increasing during this time and possibly this may lead to a drug overdose or suicide. In the scenario I have described, parents and social authorities often are most concerned about such things as school. I assure you, *if the psychological task of setting limits with clear consequences severe enough to communicate that the youngster is not dangerous is not given first priority above all else, then the youngster's further growth is indefinitely curtailed.* School is a secondary issue when psychological needs create a crisis. One can get an education or learn a skill at anytime.

Unless we have a proven track record, a child is always going to test to see if we can or will really make our "No" stick. When the child is testing us, the message is always, "You don't care about me. You don't really love me," which implies, "If you really loved me you would give me what I want—now." Obviously, if we granted their demand, we would not only promote lifelong infancy, but we also would be agreeing by way of our behavior that the child is correct. We might as well say, "I doubt I love you; therefore, I must prove to you that I do by giving you that for which you are asking!" In order to be effective, we must be able to think, if not say, "If giving you what you want has anything to do with loving you, then I don't love you." This makes it clear that we trust our love and that loving and giving in to the child's desires are not connected.

Usually, when I try to answer the question asked by parents, "Give me some specific examples of consequences?" I ask, "What does the child like or enjoy the most?" I next ask, "What would you most hate to take away?" and then proceed with "What was the first thought that crossed your mind?" A mother might respond immediately with "I couldn't do that, I couldn't spank him." The father that is coaching his son's ball team may admit that kicking him off the team is what he would most dislike to do. Someone else might say, "Take him out of Cub Scouts, but he loves it and it is so good for him. It is the only thing in which he really shows an interest besides television."

Many parents have serious difficulty thinking of various restrictions. Some suggested consequences are in the following list. Each consequence is to be increased in duration if the child protests too much:

1. Earlier bedtime

2. Stay in room for one hour

3. Take away toys with the favorite one taken first

4. Cannot play home video games for a period of time

5. No friends over and no spending the night with a friend for one week or one month

6. Cannot ride bike for a period of time

7. No Saturday morning cartoons

8. Restricted or no telephone use

9. Grounding

10. Earlier Curfew

11. Taking away favorite clothing for some period of time

12. If something special is coming up, it is most likely the source of overstimulation and it may be necessary to take it away

13. No birthday presents

14. No Christmas presents

15. Delay obtaining driver's permit, drivers education, or driver' license.

Many of these consequences may seem outrageously harsh, but in the case of taking away Christmas presents, the results were dramatic and immediate in both instances where this was recommended.

If a child knows ahead of time that getting a speeding ticket or running a stop sign will cause him/her to be unable to drive for a period of six months, then if that youngster brings that consequence upon self, he/she needs it. The consequences may well save the young person's life and prevent severe behavioral difficulties for his/her remaining life span.

When a youngster has been behaving well and asks for a special privilege such as a trip or a concert, I commonly reply with, "You are doing well and there is no reason that you cannot do this. If your behavior between now and the event indicates you cannot handle it, I will revoke permission immediately." This response often will help the adolescent to be able to tolerate the stimulation and maintain control.

Children should never receive consequences for masturbation, thumbsucking or toilet training problems. The earlier a child shows interest in the genitals the better. Peer pressure will deal with thumbsucking. Unless we are trying to train the child quite early, for example, before eighteen months of age, when we help the child with controls in the way I have described, the toilet training problems will eventually decrease unless a physical problem exists which the pediatrician can check out. This is sometimes the case.

We must not protect the child from consequences. When we remind the child to do chores, to do homework or nag to see that he/she is not tardy, we then avoid the whole process that fosters growth. Also very importantly we must not hug or reward the child after imposing consequences. This is like saying, "When I punish you I don't love you." This is very confusing to the child, but he soon learns to ask for and expect reassurance. Even with pets we do not reward them after consequences.

SCHOOL DISCIPLINE

The principles I have outlined will carry directly into schools. Teachers and administrators can expect that more of a need for helping students with controls will occur before holidays, especially Christmas, special events, and all vacation periods. When they deal with a child with severe behavior problems, predictably one or both parents will call or present themselves at school with outrage, threatening a lawsuit. They are really saying if you are going to help our child, we also need your help. They are testing to see if the limit will remain firm. Their child most likely would not have this problem if they did not also have the problem. The administrator must be able to say, "If you want to bring suit, do so!" This will actually greatly decrease the odds of an eventual lawsuit.

CRIME

When we apply these principles to societies' behavior problems, we understand why those people who have internalized no controls cannot tolerate the stimulation of simple freedom. They must repeat an offense just before or after release from prison. Those who have internalized some controls may do reasonably well on parole but will tend to repeat their chosen offense just before or after the parole is terminated. Counseling with strict attention paid to time, attendance, and money, if the person is on parole, can be of great benefit if the counselor lives and works by the rules of limits and discipline as outlined in this book. Of course, the most effective long-term pathway toward reducing crime and prison populations is by means of changing our child-rearing practices.

Our society is currently spending a great deal of money and energy trying to protect people from alcohol and drug abuse. In principle these energies treat people as though they are not responsible for their behavior, thus success is unlikely. Energies spent in the direction of tough consequences for users, would be more effective. For example, if a driver's license was suspended for two years upon conviction for driving under the influence, alcohol and drug abuse would surely be reduced. Of course, to do so would necessitate eliminating plea bargaining that so frequently results in a lesser charge of reckless driving.

In summary, by administering consequences we can reduce the stimulation in the pleasure center so that control can be regained. Tough consequences are reassuring as to one's strength and adequacy. We cannot trust an authority which is unable or unwilling to do the job.

CHAPTER 13

ABOUT DATING, DRINKING, CARS, AND COLLEGE

GUIDELINES FOR DATING

Many children are pushed prematurely toward adult sexuality by dances and dates being arranged at ages prior to or during the early stages of the body's physical changes. When girls are awkwardly wearing false breasts and high heels and boys are escorting girls much taller even without heels, it is often confusing and bewildering. At the very time when they are having an extremely difficult time adjusting to nature's changes, they are treated by parents and schools as though they are supposed to be something they are not. The result is children trying to be something they cannot be, thus reinforcing any insecurity, doubt and feelings of inadequacy.

These are times when romantic feelings are very strong, but often the youngster feels more helplessness in the face of romantic stimulation than mastery. Girls may feel like they will faint or die, "If he knew," or, "If he touched me." Boys may feel like, "I will melt in my shoes." The blushing, giggling, and stumbling when smiles are exchanged are evidence of this.

In the best interest of the child and parents some clear guidelines are essential for dating. My experience has been that parents are frequently relieved when they hear the ones I suggest. Group dating should be allowed by those who wish to do so at age thirteen or fourteen. By group dating, I mean several youngsters going to a movie, or out to a meal together, as in one parent's van or with one parent taking and another picking up. I say wish to because I do not feel children should be encouraged or pushed. Nature will take care of this when they are emotionally ready and if they are not ready, the results can be disastrous. Well meaning parents and teachers arranging dates for shy, less attractive youngsters, or those who relate poorly nearly always results in a miserable evening. I know of a prom night example of the girl remaining in the bathroom crying almost the entire evening and the bewildered boy, feeling rejected, being lectured and scolded by a teacher the following Monday for the terrible way he had treated the girl. He had no earthly idea about what the teacher was talking.

Double dating is appropriate at fifteen, or in the tenth grade, and single dating is at sixteen. Youngsters should not be allowed to date others who are more than two grades behind or ahead while in high school. Amazingly enough, this makes the teenagers more comfortable although they may argue some at first. With guidelines established the youngster very easily can say I am not allowed to date. Without guidelines, the youngster is often at a complete loss when approached.

These guidelines for boys are helpful when it comes to dating older or much younger girls. The boy in high school dating a much younger girl not infrequently has more than his share of doubts about his adequacy as well as mistrust of the opposite sex. With guidelines clearly discussed and established early on, coping is made easier in a very difficult part of development. Many parents worry about their children because they are not dating, or not dating enough. These are often parents who began dating late themselves. Of course, they wish everything to be or appear ideal for their children. Many do not realize that often boys date very little, if at all, before the end of high school. Also, early dating and steady dating for long periods in high school are a reflection of immaturity more frequently than not.

These guidelines are not hard and fast rules. They are intended to give an idea of how to go about setting some reasonable limits of your own. I will add that the most sure way that you as parents can solidify an undesirable relationship between your youngster and another is to point out the negative aspects of the other party. Your adolescent then never has to realize, much less own or admit his/her own ambivalence. When you say such things as "Gee, he is so effeminate," or, "Isn't she a flirt?" Your son or daughter can fight against your opinion and thus avoid seeing the obvious.

DRINKING

To think that adolescents will not try alcoholic beverages is as naive as to think they will not masturbate. In our culture, where alcohol use is so common and so accepted, virtually all young people experiment with alcohol at some time. Aside from hereditary patterns which predispose to addiction, those youngsters who are the most afraid of stimulation, as exemplified by a special school prom, are the most prone to abuse.

Unfortunately, some parents allow illegal drinking in their homes and at their teenager's parties. Some go so far as to furnish the alcoholic beverages for such parties. Just as with pre-legal driving, the message is, "You are above the law." The parents who allow such behavior obviously have problems in saying, "No." They may laugh at abuse unless a Driving Under the Influence citation, an automobile accident, or a death occurs.

If parents do not encourage drinking, when a youngster does drink, he/she will ask for help with controls by coming in with slurred speech, or by leaving evidence such as a beer can in the car. If the parents fail to provide severe consequences, they invite more frequent and more severe abuse. Major consequences such as no recreational driving and grounding for a period of weeks are in order.

If a youngster develops a severe drinking problem and requires a rehabilitation program, I assure you the rehabilitation staff will be very tough if the program is one that is effective. If the parents are not helped to be tough, as a part of the treatment, then odds are very high that the problem will return when the young person returns home.

CARS

Automobiles are an extremely significant part of our reality and of our inner emotional lives. Evidence for this is in our dreams where they commonly appear symbolizing our bundle of life's energy going down our life's road, or stalled, or off the road in a ditch, or wrecked.

The freedom and status of a car is the heart's desire of the American teenager. Virtually all are consciously eager to drive and eager to have their very own. Indeed many, if not most, middle class youngsters feel quite deprived if they do not have one at age sixteen. Far too many are allowed to drive illegally at age fourteen or fifteen. Recently in my own neighborhood a fifteen year-old girl was driving her parent's jeep, which turned over, and a fourteen year-old passenger was killed. The driver was seriously injured. Driving in itself is overstimulating to a child, which is why many bright and capable youngsters delay taking or fail the driving test several times.

In many ways parents unknowingly behave quite destructively when dealing with this issue. When they allow driving before it is legal, their behavior is saying that their youngster is above the law. The law just applies to other people.

If children of fifteen and one-half years are not asking to get a driver's permit, and not asking to practice driving if they have a permit, then a very important procedure is to wait until they do. A lot of unconscious, if not conscious, fears are around driving. Grave sequelae may occur if we do not respect this. The power and freedom of driving can be so overstimulating that grades fall off even several months prior to age sixteen.

Remarkably frequent the car which the family already owns is undesirable when it is designated for an adolescent nearing driving age. The preferred choice is some other car which is either just out of reach or out of the question. Translated, this means, "I'm not yet ready to have a car of my very own!"

When parents insist on giving a youngster a car and ignore behavioral messages such as speeding tickets, or accidents, the results are not uncommonly severe physical injury or death. Many examples could be provided from my professional as well as non-professional life. Parents repairing a severely wrecked car and turning it immediately back to the adolescent or buying a new one is almost the same as handing back a gun and saying, "Go ahead and kill yourself." An extended period without driving is in order.

COLLEGE

A youngster's college choice *generally* will be determined by his/her maturity as reflected by tolerance for separation, in spite of particular talents or degree of intellect. Not uncommonly Merit Scholars look at several prestigious schools, but end up going to a college close enough to go home on weekends. Subtle manifestations of the fear of leaving home and growing up are delays in taking necessary pre-admission tests and delays in getting applications filled out or mailed. Parents who remind or press are not being helpful. The consequences of these delays help the youngster admit and face the fear. If parents help, the fear can be denied. Depression in parents and in children is common during the last year of high school and the first year of college. Sometimes the youngster exhibits behavior problems, drinking, drug use, failing grades, or dropped courses.

Parents still have leverage to help with controls through economic power during college. I have developed some guidelines over the years that most parents find helpful. It is very important that the student live on a monthly allowance and not get money on demand. A full academic course load, that is, fifteen hours or more, is required. If less hours are required, the parent's behavior is telling the student he/she is inadequate. If a semester grade of below "C" is obtained or a course dropped too late to pick up another, the student must still take a full load the next semester, but pay for that percentage of full support out of his/her own pocket. This must come from savings or earnings. By full support, I mean room, board, tuition and allowance. For example, if three of fifteen hours were failed, then the student would be required to furnish one fifth of his/her support the next semester. If the student could not manage, then he/she would be required to drop-out and work until enough had been saved to return to school.

These guidelines are designed to promote growing up. If the young person fails to mature, his or her education will be of limited benefit if it is obtained. A person who has worked for a semester or a year is usually much more industrious after return to school.

To summarize, youngsters have varying degrees of fear of adulthood. This becomes manifested in lessened inner controls and resulting difficulty in functioning at their level of ability. The lack of performance reinforces doubt and insecurity. Very tough consequences are necessary to communicate that they can make it in spite of what they think and feel.

SECTION IV

CLOSURE: ULTIMATE LIMITS

CHAPTER **14**

LETTING GO

Every therapist eventually recommends to most patients that they "let go." Patients respond repeatedly with "What does that really mean?"

One must first understand that our relative ability to "let go" is conditioned over a lifetime. Those people who have a very difficult time letting their hair down or loosening up have a relatively low tolerance for pleasure or pain. In view of this, one can understand that just because people learn what "letting go" means, what follows will not necessarily translate into being able to do it in a short period of time, no matter how much they may wish to do so.

"Letting go" includes many things, such as physical evidence of difficulty in "letting go." A common example is voice problems, such as a person who makes tight or tense sounds regardless of the words being said. Other indications are stuttering or halting speech, in addition to sentences without any deflection in voice at the end which indicate closure to the sentence or statement. Avoidance of the word goodbye is a common sign as with, "See ya," or, "So long." Other physical expressions include chronic or intermittent tendency toward constipation or generalized muscle tension accompanied by headache or backache and muscle cramps, especially during sexual intercourse. Obviously, these symptoms can be from other causes, but the inability to "let go" is a primary source for them.

I have found that people who develop certain arthralgias and arthritides, as well as diseases known as the connective tissue diseases, have a great deal of problems with "letting go."

Difficulty with "letting go" displays itself in emotional evidence. People hold back emotionally. The more their feelings are stimulated, the more they tighten up or withdraw emotionally, if not physically. They will avoid anger, tears, surprises, or excitement. Conversely, they often pretend feelings to cover their fear of genuine emotion. Examples might include many movie stars, ministers, salesmen, and politicians who stage the expression of emotion.

People's degree of distress at losing games, money, making mistakes or admitting weakness or faults, even the ability to say, "I don't know," reflects a relative difficulty "letting go." Those who store things even though they are worn out or no longer used, who are "pack rats" with their attics and garages filled, closets stuffed, and all space under the beds used have trouble "letting go." The opposite manifestation would be people who never keep anything unnecessary. Everything they have must appear clean, in order, or even sterile, at all times.

All of these examples are **expressions** of, or **defenses** against facing the pain of separation. Now I hope that what is rather obvious from these examples is that these people would all be relatively overprotective and would have much difficulty forming close attachments as well as tolerating separation from any other persons even if temporary. Even many therapists or counselors do not really know the monumental task they are recommending when they use the simple words, "You must let go!"

Extreme examples of "letting go" problems result in children of age forty still living at home with mother, having never learned to drive, hold a job, or take the risk of involvement with the opposite sex. It may also result in a person who keeps pets when the pets have lost nearly all bowel and bladder control; the rugs and baseboards of the house are ruined, and the air in the house is so malodorous as to keep all people other than the owner outside. I have seen patients who represent such extremes.

Frequently people have more difficulty "letting go" after reaching adulthood than when they were younger, because as their dreams come true in the form of career, spouse, home, and children, they have more to lose. I know of no other pathway toward increasing one's ability to "let go" other than increasing one's ability to risk and tolerate the pain of separation. I have found no easy way of communicating how to "let go." Since "letting go" of a certain amount of one's aggression is required to discipline ourselves and our children, through *Limits* I have certainly been trying to give you some idea of what is required.

Many athletic coaches of bygone times would say, "No pain, no gain!" One hears it less as the idea has been challenged. In the area of emotional growth we could all well afford to seal the idea in memory. It is the only path toward "letting go."

CHAPTER **15**

SEPARATION

Frequently a patient will see me for several sessions and then suddenly announce, "I'm not going to continue to see you. Somehow I know you are going to hurt me!" Early in my career I tried to reassure patients that I would not hurt them. These responses did not lead toward trust. I now respond with, "Yes, I will hurt you! The more we become subjectively involved, the more pain we are going to both suffer when you finish here and we say goodbye. If that does not occur, then you will have wasted your time and money. This really means that the more it hurts, the better." Subjective involvement is essential. I believe objective, or social involvements, interfere with therapy and may lead to downright exploitation of the patient by the therapist. Any objective involvement could possibly be an attempt to satisfy the therapist's emotional needs, economic needs in the case of business involvement, or even sexual needs. All of these have been known to occur. I have difficulty believing that any objective involvement will not eventually prove destructive to both the patient and the therapist. The response indicating mutual pain does lead to trust because it is honest. I believe any other response is relatively dishonest in spite of the best intentions.

The goal of therapy, or growth, is to increase one's tolerance for frustration, ambiguity, and emotional pain. The problem is that most people believe their pain is the worst possible pain because they only live inside one skin and comparison with any other is difficult, if not impossible. Whereas a competent therapist can compare by observations, such as I have described in the chapter on maturation, the patient has only one set of subjective experiences for evaluation. People regress when reacting to the pain of separation.

LOSS

One thing is certain; we are going to lose everything we have, including our own lives. To the extent, then, that we try to control loss or live in fear of losing, we are not free. The main reason we all limit our involvement is because we are afraid of the pain of separation.

The extent to which we can tolerate involvement determines how much we can allow others to become a part of us. When we are able to become intensely involved the inevitable separation (even if it be death do us part) compares with having our arm severed. At first it would seem unreal as though it couldn't happen or didn't happen. We adjust to the reality with time.

Feelings like hurt, anger at the loss, and sadness are all quite easily understood. What many people find harder to understand are feelings of withdrawal, avoidance, and fatigue. These are easier to understand if you think of a wounded animal in the woods. It would find a place to hide for healing to take place and only come out to meet minimal requirements. Certainly all activities would be a greater-than-ordinary chore.

Since we would be functioning without all our equipment (minus an arm) we would expect to have tremendous increase in doubt and uncertainty, dramatically increased fears of, and feelings of inadequacy and our feelings of insecurity would be maximized. The doubt and uncertainty would apply in all areas including doubt about our sexuality, our identity, and even our sanity.

It is commonly assumed that guilt is a reflection of wrongdoing, but as it applies to separation, I do not think this is true. If a mother cannot leave her child with a baby-sitter because she cannot tolerate the guilt, then it becomes very difficult, if not indeed impossible for the child to mature emotionally to a reasonable degree. When we suffer a loss, it is so threatening that we try to convince ourselves we could have controlled that loss. We say, "If only I had . . ," in order to reduce the psychological threat. The intensity of the guilt reflects one's tolerance for the pain of separation. I often say, "There is no such thing as significant loss without guilt."

The essential element in dealing with the loss is tears accompanying grief and sorrow. *It is only through genuinely letting go that healing can occur leading to feelings of renewal and rejuvenation.* The length of time for this to take place varies with the personality and maturity of the individual. (Poarch, 1986a, p.45)

People experience this phenomenon before, during, and after temporary separations from parents, children, and mates. They also experience it when they lose or change schools, jobs, and homes. It may also occur with the loss of large sums of money. It is severe during late adolescence on the part of the youngster and the parents and lasts, coming in waves so to speak, off and on for possibly several years. Events such as driver's license, beginning senior year in high school, and looking at colleges tend to trigger the feelings. The profound decrease in feelings of adequacy, competence, security, and energy are just a few of the things most people do not associate with separation. This is why people are so confused and bewildered at these times, often believing that something is terribly wrong.

Actually, the more intense or painful these feelings, when our children leave the nest, the better. I say this because the degree of pain is a reflection of the involvement. It tells us how significant and important they are in our lives. Unfortunately, many people feel abused at having to experience the feelings of loss as though they should not have to endure them. Obviously, this makes even harder coping with the necessary and inevitable losses of living. One teenager wrote of her loss with poignant intensity.

THE PAIN OF SEPARATION

It hurts, bad at first
then gradually declining into
black numbness
   that nothing can penetrate:
     The dead feeling that you
     could stare at a blank wall
     for hours and never care,
       not bored
       not angry
       just tired

So tired.
   I don't even want to think.
     Give me blankness, nothingness,
       a void
         Where I can just forget
myself.

Why? Where did all the joy go?
   Where did the pain come from?
   What happened?

Okay. You know that to feel the
pain You had to have felt the joy
   too or else you wouldn't understand
     the pain.
       Try to remember
         What was the joy?

Love. Loving, that was the joy.
   Having them close to you,
     a part of you,
       sharing the joy.
         Would you give that up?

The pain was born when they went
away
   The separation,
     The loss,
       the amputation.
God, how it hurt.
It hurts to say goodbye.

She continues:

At some point in every person's life there comes a time when they must say goodbye to someone they love. The only way a person would avoid that separation, and the pain that goes along with it, is never to love anybody. The first major separation from a loved one is the most difficult. For most of us, this first separation occurs after graduation from high school. This is the time when kids are separating themselves from their parents and establishing their own individuality. Consider the fact that for most kids, they have lived in the same home, with the same people, doing just about the same things for their whole life. The separation is the biggest change that has happened to them in their life so far. This change causes many problems for a lot of kids—it is a period of tremendous growth and that growth is very painful and exhausting.

If you think separation is not that big of a deal, think again. Look at all the problems teenagers have. There are more major problems in this age group than any other age group. Car accidents and suicide are the top two causes of death between the ages of fifteen and twenty-four, and abuse of drugs or alcohol is usually involved. Everyone talks about the drug problem with young adults and the abuse of alcohol, but no one stops to ask why there are such problems. The pain of growing up and leaving home puts high schoolers under pressure. Changing from being a totally dependent person is a huge step, and it is a very scary one. Kids who don't understand the origin of the pain and pressure are the ones who suffer the most. They look for relief from it in ways such as alcohol and drugs, and often it results in car accidents or suicide.

There are other effects from the separation. Ask yourself, "How many teenagers do I know that get along well with their parents?" I'm not talking about kids who follow their parents orders, or spend time with them out of family obligation, but kids who honestly enjoy being with their parents because they think they're neat. The answer is probably not too many, or none. Now ask yourself, "Why?" Could it be because the kids (and parents) are trying to let go of each other and the easiest way of doing this is by getting mad? It makes it much easier to say goodbye if you are mad. The anger is a reaction to the pain. You have all heard the line of the song, "Leavin' On A Jet Plane," by Peter, Paul and Mary, that asks, "Why do we always fight before I have to go?"

Most kids going through this stage are very confused. They are feeling all the pain and fear of the separation, but they do not know it is the separation that is causing it. The confusion itself causes many problems. Say, for example, a kid is feeling very depressed and scared. It is caused by the change, but the kid has no way of knowing that. They ask, "Why am I so depressed, what is wrong?" and they become scared because they think they are "different" or "weird" for being depressed. They wonder, "Am I going crazy," when actually, the depression that they are feeling is very natural, considering all the change they are going through.

Not knowing why they are feeling the strange emotions is what causes many problems. Understanding the cause of the pain and the "I really don't care" feelings toward life will help tremendously. Just knowing that there is a reason behind all the weird feelings helps because it gives some form of overall meaning to the situation. I am not saying this will take away the pain from separation. Nothing can do that. I am saying that knowing what is happening is good for both the kid and the parents.

You may wonder how I, a high schooler myself, can know about this separation. It is quite simple really. My father is a psychiatrist, so problems and patterns of emotions are discussed a great deal in my home. Also, I have observed my two older brothers going through the separation. As I go through high school, I see how it affects my friends, and, of course, I experience the pain as well. In fact, recently I have felt the separation more acutely than most because in February I received a scholarship to spend a year in West Germany. This is a great honor for me, but it has also meant that I have had to deal with leaving home a year early. When I tell you that leaving home and saying goodbye to your parents, friends and way of life is painful, and a little scary, I speak from experience. It feels like I am becoming a pro.

I realize that I have given you only one side of the separation: the pain. Now, I must also say that the advantages that come from it are equal if not greater than the pain. Because kids have no choice but to deal with the pain of change, they grow. They become individuals who can survive on their own without being dependent on mom. There is no substitute for separation to help people grow. It is painful, but if you go through the pain, you will come out on the other side a stronger and more aware person with a higher tolerance for pain and happiness, because you cannot increase one side without increasing the other.

Remember this: those old feelings that you sometimes feel, the depression, the major blues: all of us must feel these emotions at some time. It is the price we pay for growth. (Poarch, 1986b, pp. 25-26)

Now we come to the certain final separation, "Death do us part!" The question is not if, but when? As long as the health care profession is dealing in the realm of helping people to be healthy or to restore health, I see this as performing their task. The profession has more and more taken upon themselves the grandiose and godlike endeavor of extending life beyond its natural limits at both ends of the lifespan.

In regard to the birth end of the spectrum, in 1970 a fetus could be saved at about thirty weeks of age. By 1980, this had changed to twenty-seven weeks. Currently, the life of a fetus that has survived in the womb for just twenty-five weeks can be sustained in an artificial setting. Thus, we ironically have abortion upon request while trying at the same time to create better artificial environments outside the womb to preserve younger and younger fetuses. We realize at the same time that the earlier the fetal age the greater the odds that the child will not be as physically and mentally healthy as a full-term baby.

In regard to the aged, we warehouse more and more people in nursing homes and transport them back and forth to hospital intensive care units, usually several times in the last few months of life. Most have multiple chronic illnesses prior to death and are given a staggering number of pills and capsules each day and night. To others an almost unspeakable statement for them to utter would be "I wish to die" especially to the medical personnel, much less the family, lest the latter feel unloved. Are they suffering an artificially prolonged life so that the rest of us can try and avoid the pain of loss and fear of death? As Richard Lamm (1985) has posed the question, "Are we really prolonging life, or the process of death?"

I have shared the misery and depression professionally and personally. My sister was one month short of seventy-five when she died. She was an invalid the last years of her life and was hospitalized numerous times. At the time of her death, she had high blood pressure, severe heart and kidney disease, diabetes, and was jaundiced due to cancer of the liver. On the day of her death, she was in an intensive care unit. Death was predicted, but her daughter was asked if resuscitation was desired. Shocked and paralyzed by the question, she said she would discuss it with her father who was not present at the moment. In the meantime, my sister's heart arrested and it was restarted. Her breathing was then maintained through a tube in her windpipe like the ones used during surgical anesthesia. She remained in coma until her heart stopped again many hours later. On entering this scene I wanted to scream, "Cut out this fiasco!" Everyone involved knew better. The question is, Why this travesty?

At the age of ninety-one after having been widowed for over thirty years, my mother developed acute distress in breathing and requested my brother take her to the hospital. The medical team discovered that she had multiple small emboli in the small vessels of her lungs. She was in and out of coma for several days. The family was consulted regarding resuscitation and requested that there be none. We all assumed death was imminent and were accepting of this. Without consultation, Mom was placed on anticoagulants, or blood thinners, and eventually recovered enough to be moved to a nursing home. I questioned the treatment, because my mother was already quite feeble, requiring the use of a walker, and could hardly see or hear. After several months she eventually recovered enough to return home, but did so against medical advice. I spent enough time in the nursing home to tell you that the depression of the residents was so intense that it was difficult to breathe when you entered the door.

At age ninety-four, after having spent most all her time dozing in a chair fervently praying, "God, take me home," Mother fell and broke her hip. She had severe post surgical delirium, but was eventually moved to a second nursing home. Later, she required a second surgery because the fracture failed to heal. In the several months before her death, my wife and I, she much more than I, were to spend much time in this nursing home. Again, the depression and suffering of the residents were intense and very painful even to observe. At times, it was overwhelming.

After a rehospitalization to stabilize her heart medication, my mother requested that she not be hospitalized again for any reason. At that time I placed the enclosed statement in her chart. It may bear preservation.

In order to avoid confusion and misunderstanding in the event that immediate decisions need to be made, I am furnishing this statement as the spokesman for _____'s living children:

1. Internal antibiotics: In the event that a decision is necessary regarding their use, we will support restraint.

2. Rehospitalization: _____ is now clearly competent and has requested that she not be rehospitalized for any reason, and we will support her decision.

3. <u>Intravenous fluids:</u> We are against their use for any reason.

4. <u>Naso-gastric tube feeding:</u> Tube is not to be inserted for any reason.

We are in support of medication for discomfort in the event it becomes necessary.

_____	_____
Witnessed	Signature

_____	_____
Date	Signature

Ideally, this would be signed by all living children.

At that time, she also began to refuse all medications and I supported her. Near the time of her death, the nursing personnel encouraged us to put her back in the hospital several times with comments such as, "She is suffering." You can imagine how hard it was to keep our resolve. After always trying to my utmost ability to help my mother in life, I then, with great anguish, took a position of helping her be allowed to die. I don't know if my behavior was right or wrong. No doubt some people are sure they could tell me. Certainty, in such difficult issues, is simply a defense against fear.

To die has just so many ways. Some are preferred, such as a sudden massive coronary after living a vigorous life. From that kind of end, the ways to die grow increasingly terrifying. Since death is the ultimate personal encounter in life, can we not justify giving permission to the dying one the authority to preside over his or her own ritual in it? If everything which may cause death is prevented by scientific technology and mechanical preservation, what manner of death remains? Where is its dignity and its crowning effect for a life well lived? Shall only those elderly fortunate enough to die without medical attention avoid looking forward to an eventual vegetative existence?

Defining and accepting natural limits is an extremely difficult and undesirable job, but eventually it must be faced. People who find it hard to let go and face the pain of separation will be outraged at the very idea. The task will require utmost courage. Let us live longer by virtue of living healthy lives rather than prolonging death with unnatural practices.

Each week I gave a chapter of this book to nine third and forth-year psychiatric residents. After reading this section, one said with intense emotion, "This was very painful." I replied, "It was certainly intended to be!" With the exception of the loss of our spouse, the final goodbye to our mother is the most painful for nearly all of us. Loss of a child can be even worse. Fortunately, relatively few of our children precede us in death (Poarch, 1985).

Goodbyes which may be an intense mixture of happiness and sadness are exemplified by our children's successfully growing to adulthood, and leaving the nest. Other ambivalent goodbyes are those which come at the conclusion of successful psychotherapy. One example is that of a woman I saw intermittently for about fifteen years. The effort to make an adequate emotional contact and achieve a workable subjective communion was indescribably ambiguous. Not until her planned goodbye session did she reveal that she had written poems for years. They were stored and never revealed to anyone. She presented me with a sheet of stationery which I refused to accept unless she would firstread it aloud. Struggling against great reluctance while saying, "But I have never said words like these to anyone," she proceeded:

I came here today

To say I love you.

I needed to be,

to feel,

to cry,

to see.

I needed someone who could feel,

and not be consumed.

One who could love

and not possess.

Someone who could let me go.

You have touched me.

How can you know?

I have never heard or read a more profound statement about parenting or loving. It conveys a standard toward which all of us may strive. When it is achieved, no words are necessary; we feel the answer to the question, "How can you know?"

GOODBYE

REFERENCES

REFERENCES

Franklin, J.(1987). *Molecules of the mind.* New York: Atheneum.

Freud, S. (1924). Formulations regarding the two principles in mental functioning, *Collected papers,* Vol. IV: In Ch. 4, 9, 16, 19. London: Institute of Psychoanalysis and Hogarth Press.

Heath, R. G., et al. (1954). Studies in schizophrenia. Cambridge: Harvard University Press.

Izenwasser, S. & Kornetsky, C. (1989). The effect of amfonelic acid or nisoxetine in combination with morphine on brain-stimulation reward", *Pharmacology Biochemistry & Behavior,* Vol. 32, pp. 983-986.

Kornetsky, C., et al. (1988, Sept/Oct). Brain stimulation reward: Effects of ethanol. *Alcoholism: Clinical and Experimental Research, Vol. 12, No.5.*

Lamm, R. D., Gov. (1985). *Megatraumas: America at the year 2000,* Boston: Houghton Mifflin.

Olds, J. (1956, October). Neurophysiology of drive. *Psychiatric Research Reports,* American Psychiatric Association, 6.

Peck, M. S. (1978). *The road less traveled.* New York: Touchstone of Simon and Shuster.

Poarch, J. E. (1985, August). Nightmare afternoon: The star school disaster. *The Journal of the Oklahoma State Medical Association,* Oklahoma State Medical Association, Vol. 78, No. 8, 313-318.

Poarch, J.E. (1986a, September). Loss. *Bulletin of the Oklahoma County Medical Society,* pg 45.

Poarch, J. E. (1987a, June). Love vs attachment. *The Journal of the Oklahoma State Medical Association, Oklahoma State Medical Association, Vol. 80,* No. 6, page 371.

Poarch, J.E., (1987b, May). "Our kinship with the child abusing parent (Debbie K: A Child is Bruised). *The Journal of the Oklahoma State Medical Association,* Oklahoma State Medical Association, Vol. 80, No. 5, p. 308.

Poarch, M.T. (1986b, May). The pain of separation. *Bulletin of the Oklahoma County Medical Society,* pg. 25-26.

Viorst, J. (1986). *Necessary losses.* New York: Ballantine Books.

Wise, R.A., & Rompre, P.P. (1989). Brain dopamine and reward. *Annual Review of Psychology, 40:* 191-225.

INDEX

A

Aggression 33-9
    definition 33
    fear of 34
Alarm setting 8
Allowances 62-4
Ambiguity 17-8
Automobiles 88-9

B

Blame 12-3
Brain
    stimulation 8
Bribes 70-1

C

Cars 88-9
Chernobyl 4
Classics, traditional 3, 27-47
Clock
    fights 51-4
Closeness 14
College
    financial guidelines 89-90
Comfort
    seeking 9
Communication
    behavioral 52-4
Compulsiveness 46
Compulsives 36
Concepts
    essential 3, 5-26
Consequences 56, 77-84
Control
    maintaining 72
Crime 84
Curfew 79

D

Danger 71-3
Dating
    guidelines for 85-7
    double 86
Death
    separation 103
Defense 34
    obsessive-compulsive 35-6
Dependency 29-31
    emotional 30-1
    feelings 30
    resolution of 31
Depression 36
Diagnoses
    psychiatric 25
Discipline
    school 83-4
Drinking
    alcoholic beverages 87
    illegal drinking 87
    problem 87-8

E

Expressions 34

F

Fear
    defense against 41, 105
    expresions of 41
    of closeness 43,44
    of craziness 11
Fetus
    survival 104
Franklin, J. 7, 111
Freud, S. 7, 111
Frigidity 43

G

Goal
    therapy 97
Good-bye 3, 16-8
    avoidance 94
Growth
    emotional 8, 19, 20, *Figure* 23
    enhancing view 17
    natural 8

H

Heath, R.G. 7, 111
Homosexual 41

I

Identity, sexual 46
Immaturity 11, *Figure* 23
Impotence 44
Intimacy 41-7, *Figure* 23
    sex 41-7
Izenwasser, S. 8, 111

K

Kornetsky, C. 8, 111

L

Lamm, R.D. 104, 111
Letting go 3, 93-5
    adulthood 95
    no pain, no gain 95
Limits 55-7
    accepting natural 107
    defining 107
    lack of, *Figure* 23
    setting 49-90
    time 51-4
    ultimate 91-108
Loss 98-9
    fear of 98
    tears 99

M

Masturbation 83
Maturation 11-9, 59, *Figure* 23
Money 62-4

N

No 15-6

O

Obsessiveness 45-7
Olds, J. 7, 111
Overprotectiveness 3, 13-5, 20,
    Figure 23
    irrational 14-5
    parents 56
Overstimulation 39, 43, 67-75, 74-5,
    Figure 23
    pain center 74-5

P

Pain center
    overstimulation 74-5
Pain 9, 19
    defenses 94
    expression 94
    of separation 94, 97-9
Paranoia 37
Passivity 35
Peck, M.S. 22, 111
Pleasure
    pain 7-10
    principle 7-10
Poarch, J.E. 43, 99, 103, 106, 111
Poarch, M.T. 36, 103, 112
Poem 107
Principle
    pain 7-10
    pleasure 7-10
Psychiatrists, behavior 20

R

Regression 20
Rompre, P.P. 7, 112
Rules 59-65
    definition 59
    time 60

S

School
    discipline 83-4
Self-control 61
Separation 97-108
    death 103
    defenses 94
    expression 94
    pain of 100-3
    teenagers 101-3
Sex 14, 41-7
    frigidity 43
    identity 47
    intimacy 41-7
Sexual
    relationship to social 45-7
Shyness 35
Speck, R. 35
Stagnation 20
Stimulation
    holidays 69
    over 65-75
    tolerance 73
Stress 23-6
    change 23
    illness caused 24
    trigger an episode 24
    tolerance 23
Struggle 19-21

T

Tantrum 39
Tears
    loss 99
Teenagers
    separation 101
Telephone 64
Terrible twos 38

Therapy
    goal 97
Three Mile Island 4
Thumbsucking 83
Time 51-4
    rules 60

V

Viorst, J. 10, 112

W

W. Wise, R.A. 7, 112
Women, without desire 44-5

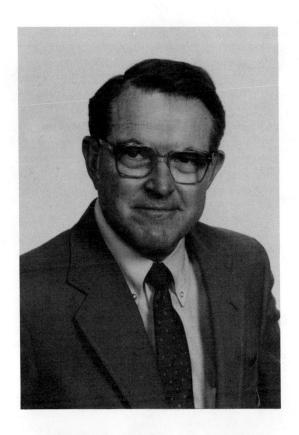

ABOUT THE AUTHOR

JOHN E. POARCH, M.D., is fifty-four years old, married, and has three children. He has undergraduate degrees in biology and chemistry from the University of Central Oklahoma and has received an Outstanding Alumnus Award. He completed medical school and specialty training in psychiatry at the University of Oklahoma. His straight medicine internship was at the Public Health Service Hospital in San Francisco. He has practiced psychiatry in Oklahoma City since 1968, and is a Fellow of the American Psychiatric Association. He is also a Clinical Professor of Psychiatry and Behavioral Sciences at the University of Oklahoma Health Sciences Center where he conducts a weekly seminar for all third and fourth year psychiatry residents. Dr. Poarch received the Resident's Award for Outstanding Instructor for the 1989-90 academic year.